About the author

Stephen Fulder's work combines writing, lecturing, consultancy and research. Trained as a medical research scientist and with an MA in biochemistry and a Diploma in Human Biology from Oxford University, he was awarded a doctorate in 1975 for his work in the field of genetics and gerontology at the National Institute of Medical Research in London. Since 1977 he has been researching unconventional approaches to health, particularly Chinese herbal medicines, and has lectured extensively in Asia and America on ginseng. From 1980, Stephen Fulder broadened his research to include the entire field of complementary medicine. Working with scientists and other researchers, and supported by the Threshold Foundation, he carried out a national and international review of complementary medicine which became the basis for a national information centre.

Currently he is a consultant to the authorities and local interests in the north of Israel, assisting in the development of a new industry growing and processing plant medicines. He is married with three daughters and lives both in Oxford and in Galilee, Israel.

D1492941

Acknowledgements

I would like to thank Penelope Cave for her valuable research assistance, Dr Samuel Reis, Dr Alice Green, Jan Resnick and my sister Adèle for reviewing the manuscript, my friends and colleagues for their information and encouragement and the many patients and therapists who have related their experiences.

I have used 'he' for doctors and 'she' for dietitians, nurses and physiotherapists as a literary convenience. I wish to apologise if this usage reinforces stereotypes of the doctor as male and paramedics as female.

HOW TO SURVIVE MEDICAL TREATMENT

*A Holistic Approach to the Risks
and Side-effects of Orthodox Medicine*

Stephen Fulder

CENTURY

LONDON MELBOURNE AUCKLAND JOHANNESBURG

First published in 1987 by Century Hutchinson Ltd
62−65 Chandos Place, London WC2N 4NW

Century Hutchinson Australia Pty Ltd
PO Box 496, 16−22 Church Street, Hawthorn,
Victoria 3122, Australia

Century Hutchinson New Zealand Limited
PO Box 40-086, Glenfield, Auckland 10, New Zealand

Century Hutchinson South Africa (Pty) Ltd
PO Box 337, Bergvlei 2012, South Africa

Printed and bound in Great Britian by
Richard Clay Ltd, Bungay, Suffolk

British Library Cataloguing in Publication Data

Fulder, Stephen
How to survive medical treatment: a
holistic approach to the risks and side
effects of orthodox medicine.
1. Holistic medicine
I. Title
613   R733

ISBN 0-7126-1481-8

CONTENTS

CHAPTER 1

Introduction

Why Do I Need to Know How to Survive Medical Treatment?

What is your experience of medicine? When you look into your memories or your feelings about it do you like what you see? Is the image of a hospital or a doctor's clinic one of caring, healing, making well, making you function better in the world, of respect, of security? Or do you feel that perhaps you are being manipulated, that you don't understand what's going on, that this is not the answer to your problems, that new symptoms appear to take the place of the other ones, that you are not healed, not whole?

All of us confront the medical world at some time or other. There we are usually alone, expecting to get the help we need from someone who has been paid to give it. But this is no ordinary service. For we are often uneasy in case we will get more than we bargained for. It is as if we paid a decorator to come and sort out the plaster work, and could never be quite sure that he wouldn't also demolish our furniture with a heavy hammer. How many times have we heard these kinds of complaints:

'I had steroids for 12 years for my eczema, my skin was like paper and I felt worse and worse, but the eczema is still there.' 'The doctor told me I didn't have very long so why did he give me chemotherapy which made me so terribly sick?' 'I had constant pain after surgery and the doctors said they would have to cut the nerves to stop the pain.' 'The doctors didn't tell me that blood pressure drugs would have such a drastic effect on my married life.' 'I've been more or less permanently depressed since my op.' 'The pills made me so tired.'

Consider some statistics:

- One person in 10 who goes to hospital receives a disease there they didn't have before.
- At least one quarter of all surgery is unnecessary.
- Two out of five patients receiving drugs suffer from side effects, in many cases much more serious than the problem which is being treated.

- 25 million people, according to a recent World Mental Health Congress have received some permanent brain damage from psychiatric drugs.
- Of 815 consecutive patients at the Boston University Medical Centre, 36% arrived because of health problems created directly or indirectly by medicine itself.[1]
- There is twice as much chance of your baby being brain damaged or dying in America, where almost all births are in hospital, than in Holland where more than half the births are at home.

But this is not another book bashing medicine. It has all been said before.[2] Instead, our intention is more positive. We want to explore what you can do to get more benefit for less risk; how you can work with the medical profession and its institutions to get better, safer, easier, more dignified and more complete care.

This book is an answer to the patient's despairing cry for participation in the process of healing.

'During one of the periods when I had decided to take the high-technology route, I asked one of the doctors what I could do to help myself. To put myself in the winning half of the statistics. "Nothing," he replied. Within me roared a helpless, desperate king: "Nothing will come of nothing – speak again!" But I was speechless and this man had nothing else to add. We sat gazing wordlessly at each other across the abyss, knowing neither of us had the strength to bridge it.'[3]

It aims to help patients bridge the gap, to cease to be inert victims subject to whatever experts intend for them, to share in their treatment and, above all, to protect themselves properly during what can become a dangerous form of aid.

There are broadly two types of patient for whom this will be of special interest. There is the patient or prospective patient who is willing to have medical treatment, who believes in it, and does not consider any other way. And yet this patient is not entirely comfortable or satisfied, and has some anxieties about possible risks or adverse effects.

Then there are the patients who do not anyway have much faith in modern medicine, who incline towards natural therapy and holistic approaches to health problems. Yet even the most natural-minded person can find himself on the receiving end of conventional medicine for one reason or another. Which practitioner of Chinese medicine is going to get off the surgeon's table if he is seriously injured? Indeed the more someone is used to mild alternative treatments, the more stressed, confused, alarmed and even harmed he may be if subject to the onslaught of technological medicine. Here is the case of a friend of mine, which first gave me the idea of writing this book.

Susan is 35 years old and married to a country carpenter, with three small children. They eat vegetarian food, some of which they grow themselves, and use home remedies, erratically, for minor ailments. Recently she developed a large abscess under her arm, after a period overburdened with work.

'I took blood-cleansing herbs which didn't help and eventually found myself booked in for an emergency operation. The stay in hospital was a torment. I felt impotent, in a health vacuum. All my knowledge and interest in natural health faded away in the bright medical world like the stars above city lights. I didn't know whether to take drugs or not; I was tired and sick and run down but I didn't know whether it was because of or in spite of them. Where were the holistic practitioners? What could I do about the rotten food? Which herbs from my garden would help me with the antibiotics? What could I do to get out of the hospital faster?'

The Medical Background

Doctors used to be far more august, distant and unapproachable. They expected patients to be supplicants, swallowing their medicines dutifully without complaint. This has all changed. The new situation is much more fluid and complex. You do still find the old-guard doctors, and medical schools are still producing doctors who are varieties of body-engineer. Yet because of 15 years of concern about the risks and discomforts of high-tech medicine, many family doctors are now more reluctant to churn out prescriptions. Patients are becoming more active. We now have a concept of a medical consumer who is free to choose, to question and to select the treatment that is in his own interest rather than the doctor's. The dialogue between patient and doctor, which used to be totally asymmetrical, is slowly swinging towards equality.

Alternative medicine used to be a hidden fringe activity, with acupuncture regarded as akin to witchcraft, homeopathy as arcane humbug and naturopathy something to do with European spas. That also has radically changed. For the first time in 150 years conventional medicine is having to move over to make room for its age-old rivals. Four out of five people in the UK want complementary practitioners to be properly registered,[4] and their numbers are increasing six times faster than those of doctors.[5] Three quarters of general practitioners refer patients to complementary medicine, half want it available on the National Health Service[6] and three quarters want to learn one or other of the techniques themselves.[7] These kinds of changes make this book possible.

Some time ago adverse effects were regarded as rare and unfortunate accidents about which nothing could be done. Today we know that they do not generally result from the incompetence of doctors. They arise instead from the philosophy and practice of medicine which requires the wielding of some very blunt instruments. Whereas previously the only option available to the patient when faced with adverse effects was to go back to the doctor for a different pill, we now have further alternative options that do not require many years in medical school. These are the approaches used here, and they can be summarized as follows:

Self Care While Under Medical Care. There are ways, some of which have been well-researched, to help yourself and treat yourself so as to minimize the chances of being on the wrong side of the statistics. You can create the mental and physical conditions to reduce side effects and speed recovery. This may include special food in hospital, vitamins while receiving certain treatments or relaxation methods to help reduce complications during surgery.

Patient responsibility. A great deal can be accomplished by employing care and prudence, by not automatically believing everything you are told, by asking the right questions, and by becoming involved in your treatment.

Alternative or complementary medicine. It is possible to reduce medical side effects dramatically by using the ancient wisdoms and modern experience of herbalism, homeopathy, acupuncture, massage, meditative techniques and so on. Alternative practitioners today give 15 million treatments a year in the UK[5] and most of the patients are refugees from conventional medicine clutching a sad bundle of failed treatments and adverse reactions. So knowledge has accumulated about how to deal with these problems, and some of this knowledge is expressed here for the first time.

Approach to Side Effects

Three kinds of side effects are dealt with in the context of this book. One is the obvious and immediate symptom which you can see is related to the treatment. If you were to come out in red blotches an hour after taking your prescription you would be back to your doctor pretty soon asking for a change. Because they are so obvious they are actually less of a problem. For both you and your doctor will recognize them and shift to another treatment strategy. Alternatively if they are inevitable, at least you will know about them and can fairly assess whether the results will be worth the tribulations. Examples of these side effects are steroids and waterlogging of the tissues, chemotherapy and vomiting, anaesthetics and confusion, surgery and scars, psychiatric tranquillizers and twitches.

Another kind are the delayed or subtle side effects, and these are of much more concern. For drug companies and even the doctors don't always notice the connection between the drug and its effects, and when they do, it is normally hard to prove. Doctors usually keep on with the treatment until it takes almost a mass movement of the public to stop it. Examples include increased candida infections and allergies after antibiotics, cancer caused by diagnostic irradiation, chronic illness of later life caused by drugs or by removal of body parts, internal scars causing pain arising from surgery, or depression from a wide variety of treatments. Often when a doctor says. 'Side effects? They're not a problem. I find most of my patients tolerate treatments extremely well,' he actually means the obvious side effects – the others are out of sight, out of mind. It is the hidden ones which have to be unearthed by aware patients and aware practitioners, for you don't always see the damage straight away. You may feel fine while taking antibiotics, even though they are exposing you to new yeast and fungal infections which appear later.

A third kind of side effect is a result of conventional medicine as a whole, and not your individual treatment. I include here, for example, the stress, poor food, risk of infection and noise in hospitals. You wouldn't have them if you went to a health spa or herbalist instead.

It is not possible to deal here with another, even more subtle, category of side effects: that of *suppression*. Traditional medicine is adamant that conventional medicine cheats the body of complete cure. By, for example, preventing fever with aspirin and cutting infection with antibiotics, partly treated residues are left to accumulate over the years with more serious diseases a possible consequence (see Chapter 11). It is quite unclear how much disease is caused by suppression. However, it is certainly something to be aware of when choosing treatment.

We also can't deal with discomforts that may result from the successful working of the drug. For example drugs that lower blood pressure can cause dizziness when you get up suddenly. This is the result of low blood pressure.

Clearly we cannot here give a prescription for each side effect with each patient. Everyone is different and needs different treatment. What we have done is to collect some worthwhile ideas and new options that you or your doctor may not know about. It is a collection of general suggestions. Whether or not it is suitable in your case must be determined by you and your practitioners. I have given scientific references, where possible, to help the patient who feels uncomfortable with some medical procedures but sees no alternative to enlist the cooperation of any doctor.

Some readers may be nervous about opening these pages, and perhaps reading about side effects that they don't want to think about. If you are reading this book while waiting for surgery, might it not concentrate your mind on what can go wrong? Might it not frighten you away from necessary medical treatment? Unfortunately there is no alternative. Because of the toxicity of its treatments, medicine has forfeited its earlier right to blind obedience. It is now generally safer to know the worst along with the best, even if the knowledge is less than comforting. We will present evidence later that anxieties created by lack of information are generally far worse than anxieties created by too much information.

Patients are better off going into medical treatment with both eyes open, being more communicative, more careful, and more cautious than before. Doctors too benefit by more open information. It restores patients' confidence in doctors and doctors' confidence in patients.

Risk Versus Benefit

Once upon a time a fundamental principle of all medicine was *primum non nocere* – above all, do no harm. Nowadays adverse effects appear everywhere at once, like noises in the mist through which medicine stumbles, while the mild remedies have been abandoned long ago. Therefore medicine has had to reinterpret *primum non nocere* as – you can do harm provided it is worth it. It is called risk versus benefit.[8] But the problem with this redefinition is that it depends on how sensitively you define harm and how carefully you assess benefit.

In this book I suggest that you do not let anyone make that equation for you. You should make it yourself and in this lies your best protection against adverse effects. You should aim to uncover the hidden side effects that your doctor doesn't notice, and you do it by questioning and more questioning, of your doctor, your complementary practitioner, your library, yourself. On the risk side go the obvious side effects – pains, itches, nausea and so on; also the less obvious – what does the treatment do to your mood, your sex life, your vitality, your sleep, your ability to solve crossword puzzles?

On the benefit side you should put a fair assessment of how your health will be improved. But health in the wider sense. Will the treatment help you to function better, to do more, to feel better or to live longer? Or will it just relieve some symptom at the possible cost of putting another in its place? Don't forget that actual 'benefit' to you may be different from a doctor's definition of benefit. Some telling research has demonstrated that there is a large discrepancy between what doctor and patient regard as beneficial. They only agreed half the time whether minor surgery was successful.[9] Mostly doctors don't take into account factors like energy, mood, sociability, sex or performance at work, aspects of life which are as important as the signs that doctors do measure such as pains, blood tests and what your cells look like.[10]

How to Use Complementary Medicine Against Medical Side Effects

Complementary medicine has been mentioned as one of the best tools to use to reduce the risk and improve the benefit of medical treatment. But what is it? How can it be used, and isn't there a conflict in the simultaneous use of such very different medical approaches?

Complementary medicine includes those natural methods of treatment left behind when modern medicine grew to dominance. They include Oriental medicine, naturopathy, herbalism, hypnotherapy, homeopathy, chiropractic osteopathy, healing and others. They all aim to amplify and enhance the self-healing capacity of the body and mind, and return body functions that have gone astray. For example a herbalist will treat high blood pressure with herbs like balm and chamomile to relax the patient, aromatic heating herbs to induce heat and sweating, herbs such as hawthorn to open blood vessels, and others to adjust the metabolism so as to remove fats. Herbalists and naturopaths will encourage vegetarianism, whole foods, fat- sugar- and salt-free diets, more roughage, and possibly partial fasting. Complementary methods require patients to work with the therapist, looking at all aspects of their mental and physical health.

The effectiveness of complementary medicine against medical side effects lies in holistic principles which are opposite to those of modern medicine. Instead of treating a disease aggressively while ignoring or even inhibiting the general health of the patient, complementary medicine would see the patient as a biography or aggregate of symptoms, features and susceptibilities which are treated together. It attempts to restore health to the whole person so that the symptoms, including side effects, clear up along the way. For example a patient experiences headaches and nausea from a long course of a certain drug. An acupuncturist will check the function of all the organ systems by examining their 'fingerprints' on various exterior parts of the body, the tongue, the voice, the skin and the pulses. He might see that the headaches are the result of liver damage caused by the drug and he will treat the liver by needles at liver points. But he may also see that the original disease, say a bronchial infection, is still there, so he will treat that too, either after the liver or at the same time. He may also help the kidney to remove toxins and break down products, both of the drug and of the disease.

In addition many of the side effects crop up in the areas which complementary medicine knows best. While conventional medicine is unsurpassed at repair of injuries, and at dealing with contagious, acute and life-threatening conditions, complementary medicine is more familiar with psychosomatic (mind-body), musculo-skeletal and chronic conditions, as well as ill-health in its earlier stages. The more subtle and pernicious side effects, which conventional medicine cannot completely eliminate, such as headache, nausea, allergies, malaise, impotence, irritability, muscular aches, confusion, slow recovery, and slow damage to liver and kidney, are signs of mind-body disturbances which complementary medicine is well equipped to deal with.

Some side effects may be relatively simple to treat with complementary medicine. For example pain from surgical scars, or nausea from drugs, can often be relieved by acupuncture at the right points. But others, such as the deformities to the patient's chemistry and constitution produced by steroids, are much more difficult, and present real challenges to practitioners. An acupuncturist cannot find instructions in the ancient Yellow Emperor's *Classic of Internal Medicine* on how to treat the side effects of β-blockers!

One of the problems is that drug side effects often mask the underlying disease. The patient arrives with a mosaic of symptoms in which those from the disease and those from the drug are completely muddled. Practitioners may, in such cases, gradually wean the patient off the drug, dealing with whatever symptoms arise on the way. This is like peeling off layers of symptoms in order to get at the root of the original disease. Inexperienced practitioners may be unable to treat highly complex drug-disease mixtures. They may have no choice other than to tell the patient to come off the drug by themselves and then come back later for treatment of the disease.

Where conventional medicine treats only the *symptoms* of a disease, complementary practitioners must be true to their commitments to fundamental *cure*, and encourage the patient to abandon conventional medicine. In these cases, the complementary practitioner will advise you to give up your drugs or other conventional medical treatments with the aid of his alternative methods.

This can sometimes create conflicts. You may be receiving medical care that is helpful and necessary, and if you have a good relationship with your medical practitioner, you may be rightly unwilling to burn your bridges. Alternatively, you may have made your decision on which therapy to accept, and cannot, will not – or in some cases must not – stop your treatment, whatever a complementary practitioner says. In fact, you should not have to burn your bridges. All good practitioners ought to respect and help you whatever path you have chosen. They should see your side effect problems as an opportunity for both kinds of medical system to work in partnership. This is why the word 'alternative' medicine is being replaced by *complementary* medicine. In fact, two out of three of all the clients of complementary practitioners still go to doctors.

Some hardline complementary practitioners will hold the view that using complementary medicine to soften the hammer blows of conventional medicine just encourages more of the same. However, they forget that only 10% of the adults of Western countries go to complementary practitioners. If more patients went for help with side effects, more would experience complementary medicine for themselves, and be able to have a free choice of treatment thereafter. Some hardline doctors might be concerned for the opposite reason. Why should patients need to arrive at their clinic with a self-defence manual under their arm? In fact the doctor should be glad. Self-defence is also self-care. If patients can take it on themselves to emerge unscathed from a stay in hospital, or to eliminate side effects from a drug treatment, it can only reduce the costs of treatment, and medical people will get the credit! In the end the best doctors will be happy to help patients help themselves, and the worse doctors will not.

Finding the Right Practitioners

This brings us to the question of practitioners. The ideal practitioner for total health care would be an experienced holistic practitioner with a deep knowledge of natural therapy and complete familiarity with the best of modern medical practice. However at present they are a rare species, and you may find yourself dancing at two weddings – with the alternative practitioner describing your problems in terms of, say, yins and yangs, and your doctor looking at the same you in terms of bacteria. There is no simple way to bridge these words – but you can get the best of both. I describe how to find the best medical doctor in the next chapter as it is basic to avoiding side-effect problems. What about the complementary practitioner?

There has been a rush to be trained as a practitioner in the last few years. Complementary medicine is a growth industry. So practitioners vary from the dedicated, careful and competent, to the greedy, untrained and inept. Here are some guidelines.

● When in doubt about a speciality, choose quality. A good homeopath is better than a bad acupuncturist and vice versa.
● Find two or three good practitioners when you are well so as not to have to hunt for them when you are ill.
● As with all professionals, choose by reputation, qualification, experience and your own intuition.

Reputation means a word of mouth recommendation by friends or colleagues. Asking around is the first step to take. Get a few names and addresses to choose from.

Qualification means that the practitioner has been trained in a course that is sufficient for the subject. Acupuncture, herbalism, hypnotherapy with psychotherapy, osteopathy, chiropractic, Alexander technique, naturopathy and homeopathy are all taught in established colleges in courses of three to four years before first qualification. This means they need to be. Don't accept anyone in these therapies who has less training with two exceptions: (a) a few practitioners are excellent, experienced and even inspiring without having gone through formal qualifications. In these rare cases a practitioner may score so high on the scales of 'reputation' and 'intuition' that the need for qualification too is dropped. (b) People already fully trained for three to four years in one kind of medicine (e.g. physiotherapists, doctors, or practitioners of one of the above specialities) can take shorter conversion courses to train them in another. These courses must be six months to one year. Anyone who has trained for a couple of weekends in the above specialities, even if he is a doctor, is not suitable.

There are other specialities, such as reflexology, healing or massage, which do not require such lengthy training. In these cases training of several weekends is acceptable. But these practitioners should *not* be regarded as full first-call therapists. They may not be able to tell the difference between a slipped disc and a spinal tumour, or a migraine headache and a circulatory problem. Go to them for help only in addition to your main therapist. If there is any doubt at all, ask for the address of their college and check up its details in the *Handbook of Complementary Medicine*[11] or other guides.

Make sure that your therapist belongs to a professional association, obtain its address, and check on it in the *Handbook of Complementary Medicine*[11] or other guides. But do not pay much attention to letters after names, or fancy diplomas on walls. Sometimes the fanciest letters and diplomas come from correspondence courses.

Experience means more than three years in practice. A full-timer is better than a part-timer. If an early appointment is unavailable this is a good sign.

Intuition means go to see the therapist and the clinic and get the feel of him or her.

Questions to ask:

1. What do you practice and how is it done?

2. Where were you trained? How long was the course? Was it full or part time?
3. What is your professional body and its address?
4. How long have you been in practice at this address?
5. At which other places have you practiced?
6. What are your fees and when do I pay them? (You shouldn't have to pay in advance for any treatment.)

You can get your alternative practitioner to visit you in hospital (see Chapter 6). But you should get to know him/her, and be treated beforehand.

REFERENCES

1. *Whole Life Times*, September 1985.
2. Illich, I. *Limits to Medicine*, Penguin, London (1977); Weitz, M. *Health Shock*, David and Charles, London (1980); Coleman, V. *The Medicine Men*, Arrow (1977); Inglis, B. *The Diseases of Civilisation*, Hodder & Stoughton, London (1981).
3. Brohn, P. *Gentle Giants*, Century (1986) (quoting King Lear).
4. UK Gallop Poll, September 1986, sponsored by the Council for Complementary and Alternative Medicine.
5. Fulder, S. and Monro, R. *Lancet* 2, 542–545, (1985).
6. Wharton, R. and Lewish, G. *Brit. Med. J.* 292 1498–1500 (1986).
7. Reilly, D. T. *Brit. Med. J.* 287 337–339 (1983).
8. Bunker, J. *et al* (eds), *Costs, Risks and Benefits of Surgery*, OUP, N.Y. (1978); Cochrane, A. *Effectiveness and Efficiency*, Nuffield Provincial Hospitals Trust (1972).
9. *Soc. Science and Med.* 13A 347 (1979).
10. Hunt, S. M. *et al*, *J. Psychosom. Res.* 28 105–114 (1984).
11. Fulder, S. *The Handbook of Complementary Medicine*, Coronet, London (1987).

CHAPTER 2

Where It All Starts: Doctors, Dialogues, Diagnosis

Dr Franz Ingelfinger, editor of the influential *New England Journal of Medicine*, once said that, '80% of modern illnesses are either self-limited or not treatable by modern medicine and surgery.' Despite the practised confidence of doctors, the pill for every ill of the drug industry and the diverse resources offered by the hospital, medicine is only really effective in certain areas. It does well, for example, at treating injuries, acute infections, serious and life-threatening organic diseases, tropical diseases and failure of the mechanics (such as blockages). However it is not particularly successful at treating chronic or recurring infections, degenerative diseases such as those of the blood vessels in their early stages, skin problems, psychosomatic conditions, arthritis, or musculoskeletal problems such as bad backs, to cite a few examples.[1] Unfortunately doctors often won't admit the lack of success, and will prescribe drugs and treatments that are just palliative (such as painkillers for joint problems), that have side effects, and that prevent or delay you from going elsewhere or treating yourself.

So the first goal of a surviving patient is not to get involved in unnecessary medical treatments. This does not mean sitting at home stoically battling against virulent diseases rather than seeing the doctor. It means learning how to decide whether to seek advice from your doctor, your acupuncturist or your grandmother. If you take 1000 adults, 750 of them will have some kind of symptom or injury every month. Of these only 250 will go to a doctor and only 10 will be referred to a hospital.[2] Make sure you are not in the 250, and especially not in the 10, unless it is really necessary.

The second goal is to make sure that you get the right treatment, that is the treatment that provides the maximum benefit for the minimum risk. The doctor should do this for you. It is his job. However there is ample evidence that in today's world this does not always happen. The doctor is no longer a conductor of the therapy. He is losing his skills to machines, monitors and statistics, losing his humanity to institutions and losing his options to the drug companies. You cannot reform the doctor but you can take steps to get the best and leave the rest.

Let's look at a case to understand what the surviving patient needs in order to achieve these goals. A letter reached me from Maureen, a 58-year-old Oxford woman, giving a story which is very typical of people who go to alternatives after unsuccessful treatment with conventional medicine. I abstract it here.

> *'When I needed help for depression following deaths in the family, my doctor gave me antidepressants (Lentizol) and five Valium a day. I didn't take the Valium and managed to get off the antidepressants after a year, but my freedom was marred by bouts of tiredness – I could curl up on a roundabout and sleep like a log – plus a great deal of trouble with my digestive system. My doctor tended to give you analgesics for pains, antibiotics for sore throats and coughs, and anti-depressants for anything else. When I asked for help as far as nutrition was concerned he said "You're the expert with that."*
>
> *The doctor gave me Gaviscon (an antacid) and said I was making too much acid. I grew more tired and he decided to send me to a specialist. Then began a series of X-rays, barium enema, blood tests, and an endoscopy (internal examination from mouth to duodenum). The only thing they could say was I had an inflamed gut throughout. "The duodenum seemed to resent the intrusion of the endoscope." I was put on a course of Colofac. I felt better, then worse, then better, then worse, and started and stopped with the pills repeatedly. Once, while waiting to see the specialist I listened to the conversations of the other patients and they were all on Colofac and some of them had had several endoscopies. That did it! The next day I saw a homeopathic doctor. She examined me thoroughly.'*

Maureen was cured in a relatively short time and went back to see the specialist.

> *'I felt fine and was signed off by the specialist in two minutes. He just grimaced when I started to tell him about my homeopathic treatment!'*

More important, she was also guided for the first time . . .

> *'The homeopathic doctor told me that whenever I felt in need of a "pill" I should take a little honey in water and a teaspoon of brandy and go for a brisk walk of at least half a mile. I do.'*

Maureen was clearly not entirely comfortable with her medical treatment – she tried to get off her drugs but succeeded only in yo-yoing back and forth. In the end intuition stopped her slide down the slippery slope before it could lead to more harmful drugs, more tests, exploratory surgery and so on. She had the will to be a surviving patient but she had to go through much travail before succeeding.

The next section outlines qualities which would have made Maureen an ideal surviving patient.

Self-care During Medical Care

Some Ideal Requirements

Healthy scepticism. Don't believe everything you are told until you have examined it carefully. Maureen believed her doctor's view that her tiredness and digestive problems were all due to some abnormal intestinal function. Even when the medicines didn't make her better she believed him. She should have questioned this logic. Indeed she might have found out that tiredness and digestive problems are a common side effect of the antidepressants, and that antacids are not a substitute for psychotherapy.

Knowledge. As John Horder, past president of the Royal College of Physicians said: 'Doctors cannot know too much about what patients and potential patients need. People or patients cannot have too much knowledge about health and self-care or the use of health services.' Knowledge about where to go means that Maureen would have sought counselling, psychotherapy, meditation or mountain climbing, but not modern medicine for her mild depression. Knowing that to go to the prescription-writing type of family doctor for depression is like going to a coffee machine for loneliness, she would have taken her problem elsewhere.

Independence. She should have gone to the homeopath before the specialist poked tubes painfully down through her intestines, not afterwards. She should have got a second opinion, or changed her GP if she felt he was miles away from her and her true problems. Independence would lead to less visits to the doctor for trivial or self-limiting problems but a more immediate visit if the problem is serious.

Self-preservation. Since Maureen's doctor didn't know anything about nutrition, Maureen should have established a therapeutic diet for herself, using whatever help she could find. She might have taken extra vitamins during the drug treatment knowing that antacids can prevent absorbtion of vitamins and themselves cause tiredness.

Dialogue. Side effects are often the result of miscommunication as much as mismanagement. The doctor doesn't know what you really feel, partly because you don't ask the right questions, or tell him all the facts, and partly because he doesn't listen. Your questions lift the veil from all those mysterious professional decisions and manipulations, and help you to be in control of what happens to you. Your dialogues help to continuously check whether your treatment is to your real and lasting benefit.

Immovability. Doctors can be, in the end, as wary of patients as patients are of doctors. If you are insistent, paths usually open that seemed closed before. This is a quality that Maureen didn't have. Applied to the medical situation it might mean insistence on your right to know all the side effects of all the drugs, or on sleeping next to your child in hospital. Lawyers are the allies of insistent patients.

Some patients or prospective patients who have wonderful family doctors may be quite alarmed at the idea of spoiling their trust and rapport by adopting these more aggressive attitudes. However there will be many more who do not have such a wholesome relationship with a close family physician and these people are in danger of becoming medical victims. However this does raise the important question of trust. A patient reading this might justifiably ask 'How can I not trust my doctor? I am told that he may mistreat me if I trust him completely, but how can he treat me if I don't?'

Trust

Once upon a time the doctor was a dignitary and a surgeon was near to God. Specialists were always great and distinguished and did no wrong. Patients were required to be in submission in their presence and in awe of their knowledge, and the doctor completely dominated the unequal relationship. I have a dear friend, now over 90, who broke her femur 20 years ago. She was given, unnecessarily, a 'Girdlestone' operation, an out-of-date procedure which made a total mess of her hip. Then followed endless hospitalizations as they tried unsuccessfully to put in pins, take them out, repair previous mistakes and so on. This otherwise healthy lady became disabled but she would never once admit that the doctors might have erred. Even if all the evidence is presented to her she will say it is 'just one of those things' and 'the doctors were wonderful'.

All that used to work very well until the medical profession succumbed to an affliction of professional hubris. They started to believe that they could treat everything and that all other systems of care, and even self-care, were unproven and dangerous aberrations. When the treatments didn't match this omnipotence, the public began to doubt. Absolute and universal faith in doctors is going, and good riddance. It has led to a plague of unnecessary medical side effects. Yet trust is obviously necessary otherwise no one would let a doctor near them. More than that, trust is itself a therapy, permitting healing in a proportion of doctor contacts without any other treatment being given (the 'placebo effect').

The answer is: trust your doctor only when you have sized him up and know that he deserves it. This implies that you have a responsibility for your treatment, to make choices, to be cautious and careful, and then, when you decide, to put your trust in the professional skills of a doctor. This is *active*, not passive. It is not trusting but *entrusting*.

The Doctor

Entrust whom? The person who is vital to help you avoid medical side effects while under medical care is your family practitioner. He is your entry into medical procedures and he should be somebody who can help you get out of them too.

But doctors are human beings, even though they sometimes pretend to be superhuman and end up by not being human at all. They become doctors by accident, parental pressure, studiousness, greed or stamina, as well as by aptitude or inclination. Traditionally doctors represented responsibility, stature, dignity, accomplishment and learning. They had to give advice and instruction in a pastoral manner to the community. Doctors also had to be very healthy. In traditional medicine before the advent of statistics, doctors measured patients' function against their own, making their own health a reference point. We won't even mention the requirements for spiritual health which many cultures, particularly in the Orient, required of their physicians.

Today's doctors do not have this stature. Suicide and alcoholism are three times more frequent among doctors than the general population. One in 15 doctors in the USA is an alcoholic.[3] They are also above average in divorcing, drug addiction and going crazy. They make mistakes. When several clinicians are given the same cases the results seem frighteningly contradictory. In one such test doctors were unable to agree half the time on whether colitis patients were getting better or worse.[4] In the USA 5–15% of doctors are regarded as incompetent, but according to the Public Citizen Health Research Group only 1/10 of 1% were ever subject to disciplinary action. Doctors almost never accept responsibility for mistakes. They either bury them, or escape blame for failures by calling them successes. When many premature babies were blinded by being put in oxygen tents, doctors said that they had succeeded in saving them, a claim which has never been tested. It is only the frequency of doctors being sued in the USA that is making them a little less tolerant of each other's errors – they don't want to pay such high insurance premiums.

More of a problem for patients is doctor ignorance which is surrounded by an armour of superiority and authority. They don't want to tell patients about drug side effects because it admits their limitations. So they state that such honesty would be bad for the patient! It is a common trap into which all professionals can fall, but with doctors it can have lethal consequences. Doctors who strictly follow toxic fashions such as the automatic removal of tonsils, adenoids, wombs, ovaries, appendixes, ear drums or some maligned piece of anatomy without proven benefit to the patient, or the weary drugging of the population with the unholy trinity of antibiotics, painkillers and tranquillizers, are generally in this category.

So what should a good doctor look like? What kind of model should you seek to avoid unnecessary and harmful medical treatment?[5] Here are some pointers to a good doctor. He will:

● Always answer your questions and give you as much information as you request. He may not want to drown you in unasked for or frightening details but he is ready to be open if he sees you are also ready.

● Give you the treatment options and let you join in the decision making.

● Have a good deal of preventive natural health wisdom. For example one man I know had severe stomach ulceration and went through all sorts of treatments. Just before surgery he saw a 'good' doctor who told him that he should always sit down and relax completely for half an hour after each meal, for the rest of his life. The patient did this, and is now getting on for 90. He always falls asleep in his chair after meals.

● Act as a pathfinder for you, to help steer your way to various professionals who can help you. He will be well-informed enough to include alternative practitioners in his list of specialists for referrals.

● Have empathy with you, listen to you and *hear* you. This comes from a doctor being experienced in life as well as medicine. It can come from being ill himself. As one doctor wrote: 'As my multiple sclerosis became more pronounced, I couldn't hide it. I decided with some uncertainty, to share this with my patients and the usual reaction on their part was a sigh of relief. They suddenly knew I was human.'

● Be confident and calm without signs of excessive ambition, overwork, strain or exhaustion. Here is a list of signs to watch for indicating doctor 'burn-out':[6] sense of failure; resentment; discouraging or indifferent persona; negativism; isolation or withdrawal; irritability; tiredness; clockwatching; being absent frequently; postponing clients; poor concentration; going-by-the-book; insomnia; giving more tranquillizers; frequently suffering from sickness, headaches, digestive problems; rigidity; family conflict; heavy use of tobacco or alcohol.

● Be well-trained, experienced and competent.

● Not assume that he can treat everything. He will be modest and open enough to know both his own limits and that of modern medicine as a whole. For example he will tell you that cortisone is not a cure, it can only alleviate symptoms for a while, and you should seek a cure elsewhere.

● Not advise you to take harmful medication, but will attempt to convince patients that they don't need them.

A 'super-doctor' with all these qualities may not be found in your back streets. But it gives you a standard to measure your local doctor by.

The Dialogue

The dialogue with the doctor is your entry gate to the world of medical procedures. Since it is not exactly a gate into a garden, rather into an unknown passageway, you should negotiate with care. The gate tends to shut behind you – prescriptions, a letter to the specialist, a request for tests, and hidden notes in your record are all scribbled irreversibly, sometimes when you've hardly opened your mouth.

There are many obstacles to opening up a real dialogue. The doctor is a figure of authority, power and a well of mysterious knowledge. The patient usually comes as a supplicant, begging some of this knowledge, asking for help. The patient may be weak, exhausted, ill or anxious as well. Society, which is represented in this case by the doctor, expects sick people to be defenceless, fragile and dependent on others – the experts – to get them better. People are instructed from childhood in this art of being a good patient, just as doctors are instructed in the qualities of an objective, detached superiority.

The end result is that patients don't share in the making of medical decisions. Just as it used to make people feel extremely uncomfortable if you suggested that their doctor might have made a mistake, so many patients would be most reluctant to even ask questions. The father of a colleague woke up one day blind in one eye. The doctors treated him for two years, without much success. He still doesn't know why it happened and is afraid to ask in case it upsets his doctor.

Information or Ignorance?
Many doctors are for their part unwilling to give information. They are afraid they may talk you out of treatment. Retaining information keeps patients in their power. 'If doctors explained everything to every patient it would soon become apparent how often doctors simply do not know; thus withholding information has the double advantage of keeping the patient pliable through the anxiety of uncertainty, and keeping the myth of medical omniscience intact through never revealing ignorance.'[7] If such a doctor is asked questions point-blank he generally retreats into authority and states that he knows best and if you want his help you must accept his

decisions. A patient came to a doctor with a lump in her breast. The doctor wanted to book her in to hospital to 'take a look'. The patient quite rightly asked about possible alternative diagnoses. During the entire 20 minute interview the doctor refused to discuss any of these possibilities and didn't look the patient in the eyes at all. Of course this unwillingness to give information has another advantage – it saves time. With an average of six minutes per patient doctors have developed the fine art of saying just enough to make patients feel talked to, but not to go over their time.

But do you really need to know? Will it do you any good to know more about all the frightening possibilities, the side effects, the treatments? The answer is that without knowing the full picture you cannot keep some control, you are that much more the victim of the inexorable medical process. If Maureen had known that the antidepressants could be making her so tired, and helping to upset her digestion, it would have changed her treatment, and her life. Consider the survey undertaken by the US President's Commission for the Study of Ethical Problems in Medicine and Biomedical and Behavioral Research, which found that *96% of patients* said they wanted to know everything.

Besides, it is now known that if patients are given more information and psychological preparation before a medical procedure, they do much better afterwards. Researchers have fully prepared patients with all the required information, such as what will be done, how much pain there will be, how they will feel afterwards and so on. Those patients who were informed were discharged earlier, had fewer complications, better recovery, less pain and even less anaesthetic than the others who were not so prepared.[8] It is obvious, when you think about it, that people are more afraid of the unknown than the known, and more fear means more stress, and more stress means inadequate recovery.

I asked several general practitioners how much they tell patients about the risks inherent in a treatment. One said that he used to flood patients with information and give them drug literature to read. However he began to notice that if patients are told about the possible side effects they began to get them, and if they were told that there were none they wouldn't get them. So he modified his position and only told inquiring patients who wanted to know the full range of side effects, or gave them medical literature to read, and to others he would indicate the major effects.

This was echoed by a London GP who has a policy of prescribing as few drugs as possible. She said that she would always tell patients about side effects that will definitely happen. She would sometimes give patients information on side effects that might happen but only if she felt they could manage this information. If not, she wouldn't say anything about possible side-effects but would ask the patient to come back for a check within 48 hours. She wouldn't mention the least probable side effects. Another doctor stressed that if she told patients about the potential side effects, they were often very pleased when they didn't get them, and this helped them to respond to the treatment. She raised the important point that if patients are told about side effects they are more likely to obey instructions for reducing the effects. They wouldn't forget, for example, to take certain pills with meals and others before meals. 'If I make the patient more responsible for the treatment he is more inclined to deal with the side effects. I therefore tell him about the side effects but also what he must do to reduce them. It is a two-way process between the doctor and patient, each taking responsibilities. It helps me because if I as doctor made all the decisions then the patient would expect me to sort out all the side effects.'

Unfortunately many or even most patients do not get treated in this enlightened way. So you should be able to recognise and deal with a dialogue in which you are not being given the information and help you need.

These are typical fob-offs that must be unacceptable to a surviving patient, recorded from actual conversations:

'Just leave everything to me, I'll take care of it all.'
'You've done too much reading' (to a girl who asked to see her x-rays).
'I do not think a worried sister will be the best help for him' (to a sister who asked the psychiatric clinic doctor what drugs her brother was getting).
'I don't have the time to give you lessons!'
'Don't concern yourself about the details. That's our job.'
'It's thrombophlebitis, you see' (to an uneducated lady).
'I don't discuss diagnostic possibilities.'
'Better take it out now and live happily ever after' (regarding a highly malignant cancer).

What do you do with such statements? They are useless to you, part of a closed dialogue existing only to reinforce an unequal or asymmetric relationship. You should open the dialogue by a polite invitation:

'Please tell me what you mean.'
'I am quite capable of understanding you. I am an adult and I need to know.'
'I will be anxious unless I know all the facts.'
'It is my disease, it has happened to me and I must know about it and how to deal with it.'
'You won't upset me. I can take it, and I need to know in order to make the proper decisions.'
'Do you agree that we must work together to get me back on my feet? We cannot work together if I don't know what's going on.'

You *have a right* to be informed of the real risks of a particular treatment and a doctor can be regarded as negligent under the law if he fails to warn a patient about them. 'The crucial decisions should rest with patients and only in exceptional circumstances should they be kept in the dark about the true state of their health or about the treatment proposed.'[9] So says the Department of Health in the UK.

Therefore if you do not get the information you need by the above kinds of statements, you can use your 'patient's power' to tell the doctor that it is his *duty* to give you this information. But it may not be worth it. If the doctor is evasive, dismissive, aggressive, or uncommunicative even after your requests, you had better change him.

Combats and Conversations

One of the stickiest situations that can exist between you and your doctor will arise when you voice your request for, or knowledge of, holistic approaches, to a doctor who doesn't want to know. It may threaten him – all his education and training, his entire hospital experience of doing things to parts of people, the beliefs and philosophy of the system he was brought up in. If you are right, he may have to acknowledge that he has put many, many patients on a path of unnecessary suffering. His emotional commitment to his methods may be huge, however covered over by doctor's armour. It usually comes out in anger. Many patients' nervous attempts to discuss alternatives elicit increasingly aggressive support from conventional medicine. Others have actually been dismissed and told to go and find themselves a homeopath. They may have been lucky. The doctor was probably wrong for them.

Your general policy should be: don't talk about it. Don't argue about it. Just do it. You are on weak ground as a patient and you are unlikely to be able to convince doctors to change lifelong views. Rely on your freedoms and take independent actions. Let the doctors, in the end, come to *you* to ask about your attitudes, practices and health beliefs. Then use the kind of concepts becoming familiar to the medical profession today, such as 'quality of life', 'the psychological dimension', 'dietary factors'.

I've concentrated so far on a somewhat adversarial relationship with your doctor, because it is so common and so frequently leads to blind consumption of harmful drugs and treatments. But doctors are gradually being taught to be partners rather than distant professionals. The old-fashioned training in bedside manners, lost for a time, is resurfacing as a conversation between equals.[10] 'In contemporary culture it is appropriate for doctor and patient to meet as equals, with the former rendering expert advice and the latter bearing ultimate responsibility for deciding whether or not to follow that advice.' This is written in a current clinical physicians' manual.[11]

The actual questions to ask your physician will be discussed below in the appropriate sections. In general they are:

- What is your diagnosis? Are there any other possibilities?
- What are the treatment options?
- What are the risks involved in each and the side effects?
- How can I reduce any adverse effects?
- How long will I have to take the medicine?
- What will happen if I delay treatment or do nothing?
- Why have I got this condition?
- What self-care methods can you recommend, including diet or supplements?

Your dialogue should deal fully with these questions. But it should not be the end of it. For you have a better chance of not receiving unnecessary treatments if your doctor knows you. Talk to him. Tell him that you are a natural-minded person, you don't like to take drugs and you prefer preventive measures in health care. Look into his eyes. Let him get to know your life, your fears and your problems. He will see you as a human being, not a cipher. It will protect you.

Treat him as a person too. Put yourself in his position. You may find a sudden sympathy for him. He may be bored and suffering, feeling as he carries out the thousandth abortion, tonsillectomy or blood test, somewhere between a car mechanic and a lavatory cleaner. You have a temporary connection with the hard world of a doctor, but he is in it for life. Or you may share his enthusiasm and interest in people, his commitment and the joy it brings. When you see him as a person he will tend to do the same to you. It breaks the pattern of production-line medicine in which you are placed in a category and fed a pill. This contact will, by the way, help your doctor to be a better doctor. Doctors often don't really know what patients feel about the success or otherwise of their treatments.

Diagnosis and Delusion

Diagnosis can take away from you one of the most precious things you have: your sense of well-being, of trusting your body, of being healthy without having to worry about your health. A visit to a doctor mostly turns up something wrong. The doctor is trained to nose out illness and abnormalities, and this he will usually do. Now something has changed. *You have a disease.* It focuses your mind on itself. Your view of yourself has another dimension, that of an ill person. Vague feelings are now organized into an illness, which even has a name, and new symptoms appear to fit the bill.[12] To take a simple example, your occasional sluggish bowel movement, once it is diagnosed as 'constipation', requires continuous laxatives. Now you do have real constipation and without the laxatives you'll feel it.

Early diagnosis of high blood pressure is useful and is known to prolong life. But that is in those with a real problem. Those without a blood pressure problem who are nevertheless diagnosed as mildly hypertensive, which happens frequently (see below), may end up having a blood pressure problem through worry. Seventy-one people with normal blood pressure who were mistakenly told that their blood pressure was raised were interviewed by researchers. They suffered depression and they began to think of themselves as less healthy and to feel less well.[13] A tuberculin test, though notoriously inaccurate, can designate people as 'primary reactors' meaning that they have had close contact with the tuberculosis organism. They may be asked to take drugs and consequently begin to think of themselves as tubercular. People who are told that they have positive test results for AIDS virus antibodies have suffered breakdowns even though the majority will not get the disease.

Medicine today is so impersonal and technical. You are liable to be diagnosed by strangers in hospitals or large clinics. Since they don't know *you* in a state of health they base diagnosis on an average. If something strange crops up in a test you are more likely to be misdiagnosed as sick. Or the reverse – you may know you are ill but doctors don't believe you because certain tests are 'average'. Besides, tests from the laboratory have replaced some of the doctor's senses, his judgement and his intuition. Though they give good doctors more information, they are more likely to lead to mechanical treatment, and sometimes to robotic prescription-writing.

Thus unusual traces on the electroencephalogram (EEG) have led to vague diagnoses of organic brain disease in healthy but unruly children, turning them into medical cases and drugging them back to their school desks. Similar fluctuations in the electrocardiogram (ECG) can start the coronary care colossus in motion with its traumas and uncomfortable tests. A simple sore throat in a child can lead to heavy repeated antibiotic treatment because a throat culture test shows streptococcus, even though most of us have this bacteria on and off throughout our lives. A high white cell blood count can lead to all sorts of scary tests, but your GP might know it is due to the fact that you are smoking and on the Pill.[13]

Hospitals as a whole tend to misdiagnose a great deal, through tired doctors relying on test results and instruments. A study of an average American hospital found that heart attacks were misdiagnosed in almost *half* of all cases. In general misdiagnosis is thought to contribute to 10% of all patient deaths in hospital (see Chapter 4).

Not only do the tests replace sound, sensitive clinical judgement, they are also wrong in an alarming number of instances. The Centre for Disease Control in Georgia, USA, checked laboratories all over the country and found that wrong results were obtained in about one quarter of all tests.

As many as 10–12% of healthy specimens were reported to be diseased, causing a train of subsequent medical treatments. In the UK, of 200 patients with abnormal tests, only two thirds had the same result on retesting elsewhere – the rest were quite normal. And in the event only three out of the 200 later developed the disease indicated by the abnormal reading.[15]

Six years ago a 19-year-old girl of my acquaintance in the Women's Auxiliaries – call her Jackie – thought she might have got pregnant. The lab sent back a positive report but her army doctor couldn't confirm it so he sent her to the hospital in case she had an ectopic pregnancy (a dangerous condition where the foetus grows outside the womb). The hospital whisked her upstairs for a laparoscopy (inspection of the abdomen through a surgically inserted tube) under general anaesthetic. Her lungs collapsed, her heart stopped, and the anaesthetists and doctors had to fight for her life. She was under anaesthetic for 11 hours, and in intensive care. Thankfully she recovered relatively quickly and went home. Two weeks later she received a letter from the hospital: sorry, this was a laboratory error, the original test was negative. Incredibly the same thing happened a month later to a friend of hers who had received a positive pregnancy test from the same lab. The hospital was just about to do a laparoscopy to check for an ectopic pregnancy when she reminded them of Jackie's case – they had already forgotten. 'Oh!' said the doctor, 'yes, we had better check the lab test, hadn't we?' Again it was an error.

Blood pressure readings can jump into the abnormal range just because the person is visiting the doctor. A study of 48 patients, reported in *The Lancet*, showed that in every case their blood pressure shot up by about one quarter at the beginning of a visit.[16] Doctors are now becoming aware of this and take readings at the beginning and end of the consultation. However they don't usually know that just talking makes blood pressure rise in virtually everyone, sometimes by almost 50%.[17] In case the raised blood pressure leads to an electrocardiogram, it is worth knowing that the trace can vary by about 20% because of the time of day. In case the ECG leads to coronary angiography, a final test before surgery, it is worth knowing that angiographers often misread the X-rays. One study in which the hearts of deceased patients were compared with their previous angiography reports found that two thirds were in error![18]

How to Avoid the Consequences of Unnecessary and Mistaken Diagnosis

Go into diagnosis with eyes open. It is not a risk-free, take-it-or-leave-it situation. Here are some basic guidelines to protect you:

● Be sceptical about any diagnosis of illness or abnormality that you don't already feel, especially if the diagnosis is based on lab tests. Ask for a repeat of any abnormal tests, if possible in another lab. But wait a while for your second test. Sometimes abnormal readings are correctly identified by the lab but are due to a passing phenomenon.

● Remember that diagnosis should clarify symptoms you have, not make you look for those you don't have.

● Rely on an experienced general practitioner whom you trust, who knows your history and who knows you, more than on strangers, however qualified they may be. A good GP will carry out a series of tests when you are healthy so as to have a baseline in case you are sick. He should ask for repeats of abnormal lab tests as a matter of course.

● If lab tests and diagnosis show that you have the beginnings of a health problem such as 'pre-diabetic' or 'mild hypertension' treat it as a warning. Seek treatment from *complementary medicine*. Nutritional, natural-preventive, traditional, herbal, homeopathic and oriental treatments all work well at the early stages of diseases, whereas conventional medicine does not. The drugs prescribed for pre-diabetes, raised cholesterol or mild hypertension carry much risk and little benefit, and any lifestyle advice your doctor gives you will have been learnt from natural therapists anyway.

● Don't be afraid to request a second opinion if your doctor advises more serious tests (such as laparoscopy, cardiac catheterization, cytoscopy or barium gastro-intestinal X-ray series) on the basis of lab tests for a condition which you do not feel. Take the lab tests with you but respect the second-opinion doctor's wish to do his own.

● Keep minor symptoms to yourself. Unless symptoms are serious, unusual for you, persistent or possibly related to some serious disease in the history of your family or yourself, don't run straight off to get a diagnosis. Treat a headache which you feel is a tension headache with a hot bath, a rest, a massage; treat a sore throat with lemon and honey; treat insomnia wih herb teas of chamomile, lemon balm, or valerian; treat an autumnal fever with fluids, rest and cold water compresses.

● Don't be continually diagnosed because you are worried about having a disease but there are no signs of it. Doctors can easily give you much more to worry about.

● When you undergo an invasive test such as a biopsy or catheterization ask that you be shown the results and discuss them before further medical steps are taken. Do not sign a consent form to 'other measures that may be necessary'. Only permit the test itself.

Mass Screening

Screening of the whole population is a natural extension of preventive medicine, and used to be much advocated. It is hard to argue against the concept of testing everyone in order to catch disease early. But some did, in particular the eminent Professor Archibald Cochrane, and received a great deal of hostility for their pains. Of course it does catch some diseases early, but it also enters many people into medical treatment unnecessarily. Prevention should keep people away from their doctor, screening collects them for the doctor. For every case of a disease that is caught early there is a case of a disease that is treated when it would have got better by itself, and a case of a healthy person treated or biopsied because the screening test gave a wrong result. The net result is that a screened group of people is no more healthy, has no fewer diseases, has the same amount of hospitalization and the same death rate as an unscreened group. Several studies have shown[19] that it just wastes money, creates anxiety and leads to unnecessary treatment. A few people are helped.

For example cervical smears (the 'Pap' test) to test for cervical cancer were recommended for all women for a time, but they were found to be 5–10% in error. Many women were encouraged to have biopsies under anaesthetic or even their wombs removed because of a falsely positive Pap test. Others have had their wombs removed because of innocuous non-malignant growths discovered in screening.

Screening can, however, be useful in specific well-defined instances. Obviously it is necessary to test for contagious diseases as in the mass screening for AIDS virus antibodies. Also, it is worthwhile in high-risk groups such as smokers over a certain age with a family history of cancer, or women who are susceptible to breast cancer, provided any X-rays used for screening are of the newer low-dose type.

The same considerations apply to that yearly ritual, the annual check-up. Many companies demand it, and it isn't a bad thing in principle. But modern medicine is not well equipped to respond to the answers that arise. For example a doctor may find that you have mild hypertension and raised blood cholesterol. You will be told to reduce your intake of animal fat and salt, which is essential advice. But you may also be given drugs, such as diuretics, β-blockers and cholesterol-lowering drugs which are not likely to increase your long term health and survival (see Chapters 10, 12), and will cause unacceptable side effects. You may enter the illness catgory and feel worse all round. The 1979 Canadian Task Force on Periodic Health Examination carried out a three-year study on the value of an annual check-up and concluded that it casts the net too widely, and is 'inefficient and at times potentially harmful'. It rarely detects serious disease and often creates worry and harmful medical treatment of the reasonably healthy.

Instead you should go for an occasional check-up to a good practitioner. You ought to leave his office feeling better, not worse. Most important, you should carry away *instructions not prescriptions*. Complementary medicine gives real teeth to preventive measures. For example an acupuncturist will not just tell you to stop smoking, but will help to restore a healthier balance to your body and mind so that you gradually feel that cigarettes are superfluous.

REFERENCES

1. Cochrane, A. L. *Effectiveness and Efficiency*, Nuffield Provincial Hospital Trust (1972); Inglis, B. *Diseases of Civilisation*, London, Hodder & Stoughton (1981); McKeown, T. *The Role of Medicine*, Nuffield Provincial Hospital Trust, London (1976).
2. Pratt, L. *J. of Comparative Family Studies,* **4** 13–31 (1973).
3. Bissell, L. & Jones, E. W., *Am. J. Psychiat.* **133** 1142–6 (1976).
4. Graham, N. G. *et al, Brit. Med. J.* **2**, 741–8 (1971).
5. LeMaitre, G. D. *How to Choose a Good Doctor*, Andover, US (1979).
6. Bactey, R. *Coping with Stress in Caring*, Blackwell Scientific, Oxford (1985).
7. Bennett, G. *Patients & Their Doctors*, Balliere, Eastbourne (1983).
8. Hayward, D. J. *Information – A Prescription Against Pain*, Whitefriars Press, London (1975); see also refs. 34, 40 of Chapter 6.
9. National Consumer Council, *Patients Rights*, HMSO, London (1983).
10. Pendleton, D. *The Consultation: An Approach to Learning and Understanding*, OUP, Oxford (1984).
11. Book by Katon and Kleinman, title unknown, quoted in Hang, M. and Lavin B. *Consumerism in Medicine*.
12. Scheff, T. J. *Behav. Sci,* **8** 97–107 (1963).
13. *Am. J. Public Health* (November 1981).
14. Fisch, *et al, J. Am. Med. Assoc.* **234** (3/11/1975).
15. Bradwell, A. R. *Lancet,* **2** 1071 (1974).
16. *Lancet* **2**, 695 (1983).
17. Lynch, J. J. *Isr. J. Medical Science*, (May 1982).
18. Isner, J. M. *Circulation*, **63** No.5 (1981) quoted in *Prevention*, p. 53 (September 1983).
19. Holland, W. *et al, Int. J. Epidemiology*, **6** No. 4 (1977).

CHAPTER 3

X-rays: Invisible, Lethal, Avoidable

The Facts about X-ray Risks

X-rays are very high-frquency waves which have so much energy that they crash through living tissues like birdshot through a bush. They are completely stopped only by highly dense metals such as lead. The body absorbs a little of this radiation in proportion to the density of its tissues. In diagnosis the shadows of the absorbed X-rays are recorded on a special film. The old machinery produced a greater energy of radiation which was scattered more widely; today the equipment is more accurate and the films more sensitive. This permits better pictures, which can outline soft tissue as well as bone, using less total radiation.

A number of related diagnostic techniques use X-rays. These include *fluoroscopy*, in which the X-ray shadow of the body is cast on to a screen which can then be photographed, and the *brain scanner* which uses a moving beam of X-rays to slice across the brain and gradually build up a three-dimensional picture. Both these require higher X-ray doses. Often a *contrast medium* is injected into the body to change the density of certain tissues in order to distinguish them in X-ray pictures. The medium can be air (injected into the brain cavities), barium (given as a meal or enema to observe the digestive system) or other materials.

Diagnostic radiation causes some damage, as it bursts through, to the genetic information or central control system, which the cells use to duplicate themselves. The chances of damage are in proportion to the dose, and the observed result of this damage are cancers in the body, or abnormalities and cancer in the next generation. There is no safe dose below which X-rays are harmless. Furthermore the body never 'forgets' the radiation it has received. The effects of all the radiation you have had is stored in your body.[1]

Tissues vary in their sensitivity to radiation damage. The thymus, the thyroid, the bone marrow and the gonads are much more sensitive than skin and muscle. The most sensitive tissue is the foetus during early pregnancy.

Here are some telling statistics:

● There may be some individuals who are much more sensitive.

Asthmatic young children, X-rayed in the womb have a *25 times* greater risk of leukaemia than others who have had X-rays in the womb.[2]

● There will be 600 to 6000 cancers for every million children exposed in the womb to only 1 rad (1000 millirad) of X-rays. This dose is less than that received in an average barium-meal X-ray sequence of the stomach and intestines.[3]

● These facts are widely known. Yet a Liverpool radiologist reported that up to one-third of pregnant mothers were X-rayed in one of Britain's hospitals in 1976, while Consultants at the same hospital thought that only 5–10% were X-rayed.[4] Current practice is stricter and it is officially recommended today that even women who are not pregnant should only be X-rayed during or soon after their menstruation, just in case. But there is a good deal of laxity in practice.

The following is a table of the dose received in various examinations – and the consequences.[5]

Type of Examination	Dose at Skin for Each Film (millirads)	Equivalent Dose to Whole Body (millirads)	Likely No. of Deaths From Each Million Examinations
Upper Intestines	500	400–800	30–100
Bowels and Lower Intestines	600	300–700	25–80
Gall Bladder	770	200–600	20–70
Spine	1200–1900	100–500	15–45
Stomach, Kidney, Bladder	770	100–200	5–25
Breasts	1500	100–200	5–20
Pelvis	500	100–200	5–20
Hip, Upper Leg	1036	50–150	5–20
Skull or Shoulder	2–300	25–75	2–7
Chest	500	20–60	2–6
Dental (whole mouth)	1100	10–30	2–6

The US National Academy of Sciences has calculated that one barium examination of the intestines gives as much cancer risk as smoking 5–20 cigarettes daily for a year.[6] Even a dentist who delivers a very low dose is putting you at risk whenever he X-rays your teeth. This dose is equivalent to smoking half a cigarette every day for a year. This is why the American Dental Association has warned that X-rays 'should not be used unless there is reasonable expectation of benefit to the health of the patient'. If this is the case with dental X-rays, how much more so for the rest?

When a man I know took his 6-year-old daughter to hospital after an awkward fall from a church wall the X-rays showed a simple fracture of her shin bone. No question: the X-ray was worth it. But then there was a series of regular visits to the hospital to check progress, and each time the orthopaedic surgeon refused even to look at her without another X-ray. Healing was normal, and the X-rays were less and less necessary – a reflex of a doctor who didn't trust his hands any more.

Radiation is certainly valuable for diagnosis and frequently saves life and limb. But it is also one of the most misused of medical tools. Experts are unanimous in deploring the horrendous medical practice during the first half of this century of bombarding with X-rays the tonsils of children who were unfortunate enough to complain of sore throats. This has produced 40% of all thyroid cancers today.[7] Yet they are not concerned that 5 out of 10 people in the UK and 8 out of 10 people in the USA have X-rays every year.

Some more statistics:

● US health officials feel that at least one third of all medical radiation is unnecessary.[8]
● 50% of all skull X-rays are not medically justifiable, says the US Food and Drug Administration (FDA).[9]
● The worst X-ray machines can give 200 times more exposure than the best in the same examination.
● 90% of all X-rays were found by the US Government to have been performed without protective shielding.[11]
● Half of all X-rays give unnecessary exposure because the beam is bigger than the film.

How to Avoid Unnecessary Radiation

The harmful effects are subtle and irreversible. Therefore concentrate your self-care strategy on prevention: avoid unnecessary radiation where the benefits are not worth the risks. Each case must be decided on its merits. If X-rays are used to look for broken bones or internal injuries then they are justified. Likewise if they are used to diagnose a suspected serious disease, for example a breast X-ray to check a lump.

Certain X-rays give little or no benefits. Refuse them. These include:

● Routine dental examinations in the absence of specific problems.
● Precautionary examinations to protect the doctor against malpractice actions (which may account for some 30% of all X-rays ordered in the USA).[5]
● Examinations to quieten you or your doctor's anxiety that there may be something there. These just-in-case procedures are usually

placebos. Placebos should be harmless.

● Bureaucratic examinations for jobs, institutions or the army. A friend of mine was called up on reserve duty. He was asked to undergo a routine whole-body X-ray by the military doctor. 'What should I do?' he asked me. 'Is it that bad?' 'No,' I replied, 'but why do you want to stack the chips against you?' 'Because the doctor insists.' 'So refuse. You'll be doing him a favour – he'll have to practise diagnosis with his hands instead.' Reluctantly the doctor acquiesced. He had no choice.

Before agreeing to an X-ray, find out if there are previous ones that can be used. Around 30% of dental X-rays repeat already existing films, and doctors sometimes find it more convenient to take new ones than call for films that may be in another hospital.[5] So keep track of all your old films, especially if you move to another dentist or physician.

If a fresh X-ray is unavoidable make sure it is as safe as possible:

● Proper shielding is vital. Insist on a lead apron in dentistry; the testes and ovaries must be shielded.

● Ask questions beforehand but obey instructions during the X-ray. Otherwise you will be in for a retake.

● Check on equipment. Ask the radiologist or dentist whether the machine is a new low-dose type (these have rectangular apertures, the old type may have a plastic cone) and if it has recently been serviced or inspected.

● Protect children, especially the unborn. Pregnant women should refuse X-rays unless a serious disease is suspected. As a precaution, all women of childbearing age should only be X-rayed during or just after menstruation. Young children are more vulnerable to the cancer-causing effects of X-rays, and as they are smaller, more of their bodies will be in the spreading path of the X-ray beam. Children will be parents. Make sure that they too are shielded, for example during dental X-rays.

Some doctors will order a couple of pictures before even looking at you, so always ask what they are looking for, and how you will benefit from them, or if there is another less harmful method of diagnosis. The doctor may make light of your concern; do not be fobbed off by any of the following:

● 'I wouldn't be recommending them if they were harmful now, would I?' (Admitting his ignorance.)

● 'This picture will only give you as much radiation as you get from the earth.' (In a few years of walking on it.)

● 'With the new equipment today the risk is minimal.' (But it exists.)

You should explain that your concern is a rational awareness of risks and benefits. Your goal is to make the doctor stop and consider for a moment how real is this need for X-rays.

How Can I Protect my Body from Diagnostic Radiation?

Diagnostic radiation does not create obvious tissue damage, therefore the protective procedures against radiotherapy described in Chapter 7 are not relevant. However something should be done to protect the cells from diagnostic X-rays. This is because the radition creates genetic damage by charging up or energizing certain molecules within the cell. These molecules become 'free radicals' which means, to use an unscientific but easily understandable explanation, that they go berserk.

The body already runs an extensive housekeeping operation to catch and destroy any free radicals that crop up. Its equipment includes anti-oxidant materials such as glutathione, cysteine, or vitamins C and E, and enzymes (catalytic workhorse proteins).[12]

There is a good deal of evidence that these materials can protect living tissues from radiation. For example the creature with the highest levels of these protective enzymes is a bacterium, radiodurans, which is found comfortably domiciled inside nuclear reactors.

It is likely that free radicals contribute to ageing, and the efficiency of these housekeeping materials is one of the ways in which our lifespan is assured.[13] In fact doses of these substances can prolong the normal lifespan of animals.[14]

Vitamin C works as a general damage protector besides helping to restore cysteine and glutathione.[15] The latter are sulphur-containing amino acids (the building blocks of proteins) with a special protective ability. Cysteine is used as the traditional anti-radiation pill. Soviet researchers have tested some 25,000 different substances to find a radiation protective for their cosmonauts in space. They reasoned that an ounce of radiation protection inside the body of the cosmonaut is worth a few tons of shielding on the outside. The cocktail that emerged from their tests, which they gave to their cosmonauts, contained the amino acid cysteine, along with another one histidine, vitamin C and the bioflavonoids, B vitamins, and certain stimulating herbs, particularly ginseng.[16]

Vitamin B5, pantothenate, has been found to protect animals from radiation[17] and vitamin B2, riboflavin, encourages the liver to make the crucial housekeeping enzyme, glutathione reductase.[18] B2 must always be balanced with B6 for metabolic reasons. One more useful component is selenium, which is a constituent of the same enzyme glutathione reductase. The National Cancer Institute has suggested raising the recommended daily allowance of selenium to 200 micrograms on the grounds that it protects against cancer and other damage.

In practice you can take the following protective materials, starting several days before any of the higher-dose x-ray examinations such as the gastro-intestinal series or the CAT scan:

- 500 milligrams of vitamin C, 3–4 times a day along with bioflavonoids.
- 100–200 micrograms of selenium a day. This can be taken in the form of selenium-yeast. High doses of selenium are toxic.
- 30 milligrams of vitamins B2 and B6 and 100 milligrams of B5 (pantothenic acid) per day.
- 250 milligrams of cysteine 3–4 times a day. This can be bought in some health shops, in which case make sure that it is taken with vitamin C otherwise it loses its effect. It may interfere with injected insulin so do not take it if you are diabetic.

Cysteine is available in eggs. An egg contains 250 milligrams, more if it is from a free range hen. You could also eat onion and garlic which have cysteine-like amino acids. You should eat three cloves of garlic a day, with some greens to reduce the aroma, or without them if you wish to return some radiations of your own to the radiologist.

YOUR RADIATION RECORD

Keep Track of Your Exams and Films

Name:				
Address:				
Date	Doctor and Hospital	Type of X-Ray	Dose	Where Films Kept

REFERENCES

1 World Health Organization Technical Report Series No. 689.
2 Lock S. and Smith T. *The Medical Risks of Life*, Penguin (1976).
3. Professor Karl Morgan *New Scientist*, **82** p. 18 (1979); Hopton, P. A., *et al, Lancet*, **2** 773 (1985).
4. Carmichael, J. *Lancet*, **1** 351 (1976).
5. Adapted from Laws, *P. Medical and Dental X-Rays: A Consumer's Guide to Avoiding Unnecessary Radiation Exposure*, Health Research Group, Washington DC, 1974.
6. The National Academy of Sciences, The National Research Council, *The Effects on Population of Exposure to Low Levels of Ionizing Radiation* (BEIR Report) 1972.
7. Favus, M. H. *et al, J. of Medicine*, **294** 1019–1025 (1976).
8. *FDA Consumer* January 1980.
9. *FDA Drug Bulletin*, 30–31, November 1978.
10. Department of Health Education and Welfare, press release, (1979).
11. Department of Health Education and Welfare, *Population Exposure to X-Rays*. DHEW Publication (FDA) 73-8047 (1973).
12. Tappel, *Amer. J. Clinic. Nutrition* **23** 1137-9 (1970); Georgieff, *Science*, **173** 537-9 (1971).
13. Harman., D. *J. Gerontology*, **12** 257 (1957).
14. Harman, D., *Radiation Research*, **16** 753-4 (1962).
15. Tappel, *American J. Clinical Nutrition*, **27** 960-5 (1974); Cort, *J.A.O.C.S.*, **51** 321-5 (1974).
16. Brekham, I. I., *Man and Biologically Active Substances*, Pergamon Press, Oxford (1980), p. 47.
17. *Strahlentherapie*, **150** 500-506 (1975).
18. Beutler, E. *Science*, **165** 613-5 (1969).

CHAPTER 4

Hospitals: How to Keep Your Head and Your Health

Prison, Factory or Sanctuary?

Hospitals are unnerving places for most of us. You enter seeking help and succour. Yet within hours you are stripped of clothing, belongings, personality, freedom of action, of movement and sometimes even of speech – for there is no one to answer your questions. The hospital environment can seem like a factory – with its fluorescent lights glaring on shiny pastel corridors and bleached faces – or with some cosmetic decor it becomes an airport.

The staff may think of themselves as kind and dedicated with a loyalty to the hospital. Yet one only has to scratch the surface a little to realize that they also cause endless disturbances to patients and themselves. The patients have to cope with uncertain rules of 'good behaviour' on top of the discomforts of isolation, strangeness and helplessness. Good patients are stoical, docile, uncomplaining, unquestioning and don't take up much of the doctors' time. Staff discourage patients from being communicative, alert, active and strong-willed. Yet these are precisely the qualities needed for recovery, especially of long-stay patients.[1]

Why is it that doctors are well known to be the most difficult patients of all? Mostly because lying in bed they are faced with their own creations. As Dr Jack Geiger described:

'I had to be hospitalized suddenly and urgently *on my own ward*. In the space of only an hour or two I went from apparent health and well-being to pain, disability and fear, and from staff to inmate in a total institution. At one moment I was a physician: elite, technically skilled, vested with authority, wielding power over others, effectively neutral. The next moment I was a patient: dependent, anxious, sanctioned in illness only if I was co-operative. A protected dependency and the promise of effective technical help were mine – if I accepted a considerable degree of psychological and social servitude.[2]

It is especially hard on children. They feel the atmosphere of alienation, isolation and anxiety more than adults. The children are expected to behave like good adults in the same way that adult patients are expected to behave like good children.

The Hospital Environment

Are hospitals clean, quiet, restful, secure and unpolluted, as a recovering patient might reasonably expect? No. Instead the bright lights, chemical smells, electrical machinery and the air conditioning add to drug side effects and anxiety to create ideal conditions for headaches, migraines, rhinitis and reduced resistance. As one staff member complained in *The British Medical Journal* about his hospital 'Ever since it opened there has been a high incidence of complaints of sore throats, nasal congestion, headaches and lethargy among staff.'[3] And the patients?

The lack of ventilation keeps in all the toxic pollutants from plastics, insulation, gases, pipes, disinfectants and so on, which give hospitals their characteristic slightly unpalatable smell. Nurses can actually get dizzy and nauseous from the vapours. There is a disregard for chemical pollution in hospitals, as was discovered by German scientists when they tested nitrosamines in the rubber teats of baby-feeding bottles in one hospital and found that they were 16 times the upper limit for this dangerous chemical set in 1985 by the FDA.

There is electronic pollution from the machinery, the monitors and screens, electromagnetic fields strong enough to affect immunity. Healers, supported in an unusual alliance by industrial psychologists, can see the way that radio, fluorescent lights, VDU screens and instruments emit waves which, they say, cause hormonal disturbances.[4] The Department of Health in the UK issued a booklet called *Feeling Good* about how to design healthy office interiors to minimize all these health problems. *Feeling Good* evidently doesn't apply to patients in their own hospitals.

Patients are meant to get a good deal of rest in hospital. Natural sleep and relaxation are essential to a speedy recovery. Yet hospitals are so full of commotion that this is often impossible. The answer is, as ever, sedatives, which are almost automatically issued to patients every evening. My wife was awakened from deep sleep after childbirth by a nurse who shook her and shouted 'Don't you want your sleeping pill, dear?'

The National Institute of Environmental Health Sciences in the US found that on average, a patient in a recovery room experienced 60–80 decibels of noise (like being in a car) from the suction machines, talking and even shouting of staff, telephones and so on. This noise is sufficient to create discomfort, stress and alarm, putting extra strain on the heart. It can cause ear damage in people receiving antibiotics and will certainly prevent rest and sleep.[5] The noise in Intensive Care Units causes sleep deprivation, helping to make patients in those twilight rooms feel that they are going mad. In operating rooms the staff are stressed by noise averaging 80 decibels, equivalent to that of a diesel truck,[6] and nearly twice the limit set by the US Environmental Protection Agency for hospital noise. Babies are most sensitive to noise and it has been found that the continuous noise in incubators into which premature babies are consigned, may produce permanent partial deafness in some babies.[7]

Risks in Hospital

Here are some of the dangers, so that you know what they are. One in five people who go to hospital receive a health problem there that they didn't have before. The hospital is the focus of iatrogenic, or medically-induced, disease. It comes from:

Unnecessary surgery. In the US some 6 million unnecessary operations and invasive tests are performed each year, leading to perhaps 50,000 deaths. In the UK 20,000 normal appendixes are removed. In a confidential poll of nurses, half thought that about one in three operations was unnecessary.[8] This does not even include those cases which do justify surgery on purely conventional medical grounds, but could be dealt with safely, successfully and painlessly by complementary medicine. A review of unnecessary surgery is given in Chapter 6.

Drug side effects. The incidence of side effects from drugs given in hospital can be as high as one in five of all patients.[9] This is discussed further in Chapter 9.

Hospital infections. As many as 5-10% of all patients receive an infection while in hospital, and a few percent, perhaps 100,000 people in the US, die from these infections. This is discussed further in Chapter 8.

Mistakes in diagnosis and treatment. Of all deaths in hospital, 10% are thought to result from misdiagnosis. On average, hospital doctors misdiagnose about 15% of the time.[8]

You Can Avoid Unnecessary Hospitalization

As with all medicine it is best not to accept hospitalization unless it is really necessary. Here is how to make sure that a hospital visit is right for you.

The office or clinic of your General Practitioner is the point where the ball starts rolling. Your open dialogue with your GP should be able to assign correctly your stomach problem to your marriage, and that of your heart to your imagination, or correctly detect a more serious problem and send you for a checkup to the specialist. You should be careful, open and ask lots of questions. He should be caring, communicative and knowledgeable enough to answer them. 'I want you to go for a checkup' should be the beginning not the end of your dialogue.

These are the 10 questions to ask your practitioner when he recommends a visit to a specialist:

1. What exactly is the problem and why do you think *I* have got it at this time?
2. Why do you think I should see *that kind* of specialist?
3. Why do you recommend *that particular* specialist?
4. Can you give me any advice on how to look after myself so that the problem is stabilized or improved?
5. What will happen if I delay my visit to the specialist?
6. What will happen if I choose not to visit the specialist?

For Tests:

7. What tests are you recommending and what questions do you need to answer?
8. What are the risks or discomforts of the tests?
9. How reliable are they?
10. Are there any other ways to arrive at a diagnosis?

Take time. Tests are rarely so urgent that you cannot take time to be prepared. Don't be rushed into the consultant's appointment, unless it is very urgent, without giving yourself preparation time.

Be informed. Read about your suspected condition in health books, health magazines, medical texts. Contact self-help groups (addresses are at the back of this book). Check with them whether the consultant and hospital you have been referred to is the best for your problem. If necessary go back to your GP to ask further questions if the information you have found conflicts with his earlier explanations.

Prepare a record of your symptoms and the questions you want to ask the consultant. You will be faced with a busy specialist, behind a pile of papers, who may hardly look at you. You may be rationed to a few squeaks about your symptoms interrupted by the telephone. So have your qestions ready.

Consider obtaining a consultation with a complementary practitioner before the specialist appointment. Most diseases can be helped to some extent by dietary, acupuncture, osteopathic/chiropractic, psycho-therapeutic, homeopathic or herbal methods. Some can be dealt with so successfully by complementary medicine that you can expect to avoid all further medical intervention. (See the author's *Handbook of Complementary Medicine*.[10] Talk to people who have been to complementary practitioners, if you are not sure about it. Practitioners belonging to the main professional bodies, with a good reputation and several years' experience, will normally give you a fair assessment of what you can gain by complementary medicine. If you go to an holistic health centre you have more chance of hitting the right alternative speciality for your problem. Some cost at this stage may save you a great deal later on, and most therapists have concessionary fees for those with limited means.

Seeing the Consultant

Your practitioner will advise you of, or refer you to, a particular consultant/surgeon in a particular hospital. You should ask to be referred to a surgeon who has a great deal of experience of the operation in mind, who has a good reputation among medical people, and who works in the hospital that is renowned for the treatment of this particular condition. If you are paying then you can shop around.

You should tell him of your problem and ask:

1. What is the illness and why have I got it?
2. What are the treatment options? How do their results compare? What are the statistics and research evaluations of each?
3. What will treatment or surgery do? What are the risks? What will be the physical and psychological consequences and how long will it take to be back on form?
4. What will happen if I say no? Will it reduce the quality of my future life more than the side effects of the treatment?
5. What will happen if I delay it?
6. What will be the costs of surgery, tests, hospital stay, anaesthetist (if private).
7. How frequently do you do this procedure?

If you are not happy with his answers and you want to check them you can go for a second opinion. If he refuses to answer your questions or you become aware that this consultant and the hospital do not have a good reputation for your condition you can change him.

Changing your consultant is easy, of course, if you are paying him. You ask for your notes to be transferred, take your X-rays in your hand and exit stage left. Under the NHS it is more difficult since you cannot choose him in the first place, and you must accept a junior in the consultant's team if you are under a consultant. Your options are: to go private, to start again completely with another General

Practitioner (not advisable) or to go back to your doctor, convince him of your case, and enlist his help. He will often do so despite the fact that he may be put in a somewhat embarrassing situation with the present surgeon/consultant by supporting your lack of faith in him.

Second opinions

If the procedure is at all serious, or if the answers to the questions do not completely satisfy you, or if your own preparation has uncovered less risky treatment options, you should have a second consultation as a matter of course.

Many insurance companies will pay for this as it often saves costly and unnecessary surgery. However, don't do an automatic round of second or third opinions simply because you are nervous of surgery but you cannot find fault in the chosen treatment method. Under the National Health Service a specialist or consultant is already a kind of second opinion since you have been referred on from your general practitioner. If you want a second opinion beyond your consultant you may have to pay for it. However NHS consultants sometimes permit a second NHS opinion in difficult cases. It is worth asking.

The second consultant to whom you refer should do all the necessary tests except those that are hazardous, including X-rays, which you should bring with you. The consultant should know you want advice, not treatment, so he will give a detached picture. You should not tell him the diagnosis and conclusion of the first consultant. Don't choose a consultant for a second opinion who is from the same practice or hospital as, or recommended by, the first one.

Which Hospital?

Hospitals vary greatly. They may be large or small, teaching or non-teaching, specialist (children's, maternity, eyes, accidents etc.) or general, short-stay or long-stay with emphasis on nursing care or on high-tech surgery.

They vary in standards of care as well as type of professional expertise. In some hospitals there is a high turnover of staff, unnecessarily rigorous application of meaningless rules, a stricter hierarchy, more mystification and uncertainties for the patient, less personal nursing care, and a feeling that the hospital is such a total institution that nobody would notice if all the patients disappeared overnight. In other places the reverse is true, and patients find a pleasing combination of a well-oiled system that nevertheless allows plenty of personal contact and individual care by the staff. This is not just a matter of comfort. It is also a question of your recovery. A study of different hospitals within the Manchester region found that it took 11 days to recover from appendix removal in hospitals where the staff were grumpy and didn't stay for long, and an average of 8 days where the atmosphere was better.[11]

Hospitals don't need to be depressing places. A large new public hospital being built at Newport in the Isle of Wight is designed specifically to lift the spirits of patients. There is a conservatory at the end of every ward which looks out over beautiful Monet gardens, inviting patients to meet their visitors by its fountains, water-lily pools and secret glades. Instead of the usual vistas of pastel plaster there are natural materials – wood, wool, stone – with plants and water consciously placed for their healing power. The beds have personalized surroundings and patients wake in recovery rooms under mobiles. The Birmingham Accident Hospital is another example, this time of superb staff care despite a dingy century-old building. Here the medical staff are divided into teams, the members of which work together without pulling rank. The lowest nurse can pipe a protest to the highest consultant. The patient always has the same team. The theme of friendliness is encouraged, and even ambulance crews visit 'their' patients to chat to them. The recovery statistics are unparalleled.

When you and your GP choose a specialist the hospital goes with him. But since under the NHS you may not be able to get the specialist himself to treat you, you must pay attention to the reputation and quality of the hospital as well. You may like to know that:

● Smaller community hospitals are often friendlier, with less chance of giving you a new disease or complication than the big teaching hospitals.
● Teaching hospitals are, by contrast, better where there is a life-threatening or unusual condition.
● Some hospitals have less waiting time for non-emergency surgery (for information see ref. 12).
● You may want to look for hospitals which include some form of natural medicine in their repertoire. For example Hackney Hospital runs visualization and relaxation classes for its patients.
● The atmosphere and quality of nursing care, and availability of physiotherapists, are as important in long hospital stays as the doctors.

Go and see a prospective hospital. If you are a private patient, you can ask to be shown around. Come at lunchtime to look at the food. Check for light, fresh air, space around beds, lack of noise and smells, and above all a good atmosphere among the nurses and patients. Ask about the range of skills available (hypnosis? psychologist/counsellor?), visiting rules, use of library and how often the doctors go round.

Background Information

Here are a few things you should be aware of.

Your rights.[13] Only in the US are there Patients Bills of Rights adopted by hospitals under consumer pressure. They rarely show them to patients. In the UK your rights are governed by various laws. They are:

● You have no right to a particular treatment. You cannot demand vitamins, or a new surgical technique you know of, but you can ask your doctor.
● You have a right to leave hospital at any time unless you are mad, highly contagious or helpless and abandoned by family and friends.
● You must be asked for your consent to all treatments and *you must be told of the risks involved*. Patients must be told the truth about their health and treatment except under exceptional circumstances.
● You can refuse treatments even if you will die thereby. But the hospital can ask you to go if you don't accept.
● If you are incompetent to give consent, for example if you are unconscious, or drugged, doctors can carry out essential treatments.
● You can refuse to be treated in the presence of students even in a teaching hospital.
● You have no rights to receive visitors outside the times agreed by the hospital. (But the Health departments in the UK and US have recommended hospitals to allow parents to visit their children at all hours of the day or night.)

Your medical record. Although you have no right to it, your doctor may quote from it or let you see it on request. Where there is no other choice, patients have sometimes just taken them from the trolley going round or the tray on the desk when no one is looking. Alternatively find a sympathetic outside doctor who will write asking for them and show them to you.

Drug side effect information. This is supposed to be given to you by the doctor if you request it. However you or your supporter can go to the medical library and look it up in the *British National Formulary*.

Discharging yourself. You can do this but you will be asked to sign a form by the hospital. It may be necessary to get out to evaluate again what's going on, if your doctors and you are miles apart. One report found that people walked out of coronary care mostly because they were horrified over treatment they had received while in Intensive Care. The report incidentally recommended tranquillization to prevent people walking out against medical advice. But it admitted that the 2% that do have a very high chance of survival![14]

Too many tests. If technicians come to take blood for the nth time within a short period you can refuse and let them know that in future different tests should be done from the same sample.

Intensive Care Units/Special Care Units. Don't worry if you think you are going mad there. It is the sensory deprivation, the drugs, the stress, and the machines. Some 30% of patients used to get psychotic in ICUs, but staff are a bit more aware of it now. The staff are now trained to be more human, to talk to patients even when they appear comatose, and to soften the psychological strain. However it is worth remembering that the staff too are under special strain in those units, and try and arrange for as much visiting by a caring companion as possible. There is also a question of overuse of ICUs. Most people in ICUs need to be there, especially in the UK where they comprise only 1% of acute beds compared with 15% in the US. But nevertheless people who are in one for monitoring to watch for complications, especially coronary patients, often do better in a normal ward[15] and, according to the *British Medical Journal*, don't need to be there.[16] You can discuss this with your specialist.

The Seven Allies

The following seven allies are your patient's package for reducing the chances of infections, complications, side effects and mistakes. They also hasten recovery. Hospitals should provide them. It would be in their interest. But they will not until they become holistic caring centres.

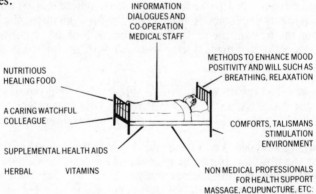

INFORMATION
DIALOGUES AND
CO-OPERATION
MEDICAL STAFF

METHODS TO ENHANCE MOOD
POSITIVITY AND WILL SUCH AS
BREATHING, RELAXATION

NUTRITIOUS
HEALING FOOD

A CARING WATCHFUL
COLLEAGUE

COMFORTS, TALISMANS
STIMULATION
ENVIRONMENT

SUPPLEMENTAL HEALTH AIDS

HERBAL   VITAMINS

NON MEDICAL PROFESSIONALS
FOR HEALTH SUPPORT
MASSAGE, ACUPUNCTURE, ETC.

The Hospital Staff

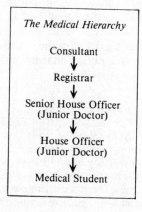

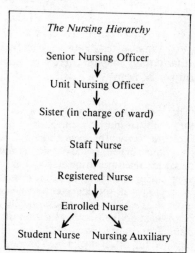

The Medical Hierarchy

Consultant
↓
Registrar
↓
Senior House Officer
(Junior Doctor)
↓
House Officer
(Junior Doctor)
↓
Medical Student

The Nursing Hierarchy

Senior Nursing Officer
↓
Unit Nursing Officer
↓
Sister (in charge of ward)
↓
Staff Nurse
↓
Registered Nurse
↓
Enrolled Nurse
↙   ↘
Student Nurse   Nursing Auxiliary

Hospital Administrators

Clerical Staff

Professional staff – speech therapists,
occupational therapists and physiotherapists,
dieticians, psychologists, radiographers,
pharmacists, opticians, orthoptists etc.

Technical Workers – Biochemists, physicists,
lab. technicians, dental technicians, medical
photographers etc.

Ancillary Staff – porters, domestics, catering
orderlies, engineers etc.

The aids complement each other. A good friend can get you supplements and good food. These bring a better frame of mind. Each of these aids is intended to give maximum life during a time of maximum risk.

Here is one example in which they were all used to great benefit. I talked to Janet Marshall who was taken to the Red Cross Hospital in Kyoto, Japan after being very badly injured in a car accident. At this normal public hospital there was a team of seven nurses on duty in the ward for 24 hours.

'They insisted on carrying out a very high standard of personal care for they said that morale is the basis of recovery. They bathed my feet and did pedicure frequently, even though I was paralysed from the waist down. Every morning either the physiotherapist or the nurses themselves gave me a massage sometimes using essential oils. Every other day all the patients had electro-acupuncture given by the physiotherapist to stimulate the nerves and tissues to repair the damage. Morning and evening they would give out hot moist bags which were enthusiastically welcomed by the patients who would place them on their body with a lot of fuss and discussion, and they would clamour for more and more. I also had water therapy for six months until I regained full use of my limbs. The most touching part was that every person, from the cleaners to the doctor, felt they were part of a team whose sole function was to get me better. There didn't seem to be favourite patients. The team worked with enthusiasm, and were sensitive to all my special needs. For example I felt at one stage that I was going out of my mind, lying there for such a long time. So a doctor came who taught me breathing exercises and he gave me a meditation to carry out to open energy centres in the body.'

I asked if she didn't have complaints. She said that she did at the beginning when they gave her drugs which she felt had devastating psychological effects which the doctors didn't understand. But they called an arbitrator who sorted it out. All hospitals have one or more arbitrators, usually doctors who have been ill themselves and so could take the patient's part more effectively in any dispute or failure of communication.

Control Your Space

In holistic terms pictures, colours, space and a sense of freedom rather than oppression are as important as drugs and drips. Your environment in hospital can make a great deal of difference to your mood and well-being, and many patients do not recognize this until they get a bed by a window and somehow find their spirits picking up. In one study patients whose windows looked out over nature were less depressed, had fewer painkillers and recovered more quickly than those looking at brick walls.[8]

Here are some things to do to improve your immediate environment.

Try and find a window seat. If you have any choice in the matter, ask the administrator for a bed by a window looking out on something.

Bring your own stage set. Pictures, postcards, posters – ask your visitors quietly to put them up. Children's wards have them but it is usually assumed that adults fare well on a diet of yellow paint!

Turn off the fluorescent lights. They bother some people and can produce eyestrain and headaches, and certainly prevent you from a healing sleep during the day. Our first child, in hospital immediately after birth, seemed to be a model baby – attentive, quiet, relaxed, feeding well – except when the nurse came in to change her. Then she became the model crying baby. Could she, only two days old, be already as upset at unnecessary medical interference as her father? We found later that it was the fluorescent lights which the nurse switched on that made her yell. Obtain the co-operation of your ward mates to keep them switched off, or ask the nurse to give you an incandescent side light instead.

Seek natural ventilation and air ions. If your medical condition and the weather allows, ask for the windows to be opened (if they do). Natural ventilation can help you recover more quickly. The health problem associated with air-conditioned environments is due to the presence of positive electrical charges in the air. High positive charges, present under certain weather conditions, cause just those symptoms described – headaches, migraine, nose and throat discharge, catarrh and depression. Negative ions, usually present in fresh air, make you feel good. They can be sprayed out by air ionizers. The University of Surrey Human Biology Department found that air ionizers reduced headaches inside an air-conditioned building by 70%. Negative ions, like fresh air, can stop you catching certain hospital infections. In one study with chickens with Newcastle virus disease, 90% of the healthy chickens in the next cage caught the disease. However when an ionizer was used no chickens caught the disease from their neighbours![17]

Negative ions can also help to give rest, relieve pain and increase energy. At a home for handicapped children, a visiting doctor who had cured his respiratory problem with air ions suggested that a large ionizer be installed. 'A survey of results after installation showed a marked improvement in children's health and happiness, and as a bonus the staff did not succumb to so many infections.'[18] Ionizers have been tried in one or two hospitals and found to relieve pain and improve rest and recovery of burn patients.[19]

Negative ions are used extensively in Soviet hospitals and clinics, and there are about 30 special electro-aerosol clinics in Germany. The evidence has the support of NASA, the National Physical Laboratory, The Environmental Protection Agency and Bart's Hospital's team on Environmental Health. Ask your hospital why they do not have one.

You probably will not be allowed to plug in an air ionizer next to your bed because the staff will be afraid (unnecessarily) of interference with their machines and monitors. Try and find a battery operated ionizer, and just put it by your bed. It is silent.

Familiar things. Bring with you 'power' objects with which you have a strong connection. It works in an obvious way with children. A psychotherapist who worked with imagery was called in to treat a boy in a coma. She asked his mother what was his favourite game. It was, she replied, a theatre of animals which all eventually fell to the ground except the frog which jumped up full of life. The psychotherapist talked to the boy about the frog and helped to bring him back. She bought a frog which was there to greet him when he came back to consciousness. He smiled at it and said 'I have seen the frog jump and now I can sleep.'

A Supportive Companion

Friend, colleague, family member – make sure *somebody* is there. Somebody you trust, who cares for you and can take care of you. Much of the stress of hospitalization – the fears, the alienation, the disturbances, the lack of information, the watchfulness for your fate – can be unloaded on to your companion. He or she can hear your grumbles, take your mind off your future, administer vitamins and medicines, get your special food, help you to wash, massage your feet and work with you on your breathing exercises.

A companion can discuss things with the medical staff when you haven't the energy and make sure you are getting the proper procedures. But what they should not do is issue *instructions* to staff in your name, as there is one thing medical professionals dislike more than the patient telling them what to do – and that is the patient's visitor telling them what to do.

A caring companion is not the same as a gaggle of visitors, who may be welcome indeed but may exhaust you with their chatting and exuberant partying at your bedside. Keep visitors to visiting hours and your caring companion with you as long as possible. The staff will probably protest. Therefore you should try to make arrangements for such a companion with your doctor. You could state that you are of a nervous, anxious disposition and a companion is needed to allay anxiety and hasten recovery. You should know that one of the usual reasons given for banning visitors – the danger of infection – is completely false unless the visitor has exfoliative eczema or some unusual disease![20] In fact there are studies showing that a friend reduces patient anxiety,[21] and this is especially the case with birth (see Chapter 12) which, with a friend to help, proceeds with less chance of a Caesarean and complications.[22]

On no account leave your young children alone in hospital. There is no greater aid to your child's recovery than you, and no greater hindrance than the gaping hole created by your absence. This has been clearly established by psychologists who see children go through the stages of screaming protest, despair and apathy (which the staff sometimes call 'settling in'!) and finally denial of their feelings.[23] The hospital loses by not requesting parents to assist in their child's care, since abandoned children are far harder to nurse. Parents also do not save anything because children who are left in hospital regress and will certainly have their own back afterwards in terms of bed-wetting, crying at night and clinging or aggressive behaviour.

Some hospitals allow parents to be with their children all the time, but others do not, and few have rooming-in facilities, or folding beds for parents to sleep by their children. However as the Patients Association comments 'the mother with an air-cushion, vacuum flask, knitting and determination can usually manage to sit up at night by the child's bed if she quietly makes up her mind to do so.'[24] The Department of Health and Social Security in the UK, the National Institute of Mental Health, and the American Medical Association all strongly recommend that hospitals encourage parents to stay with their children, so you have some backing against inhuman hospital visiting rules where you encounter them.

Understanding Stress and Anxiety in Hospital

You may feel you are going a bit crazy in hospital. But you will not be alone. Other patients feel the same although they may not talk about it. Research has shown that most people feel quite a lot of anxiety as soon as they enter. This can even be measured by monitoring the alarm hormones circulating in the blood. They increase as soon as you walk through the door of the hospital and can stay high thereafter.[25] Anxiety and disorientation during a hospital stay may be due to the strangeness, lack of information, the alienation, the lack of contact with the staff, the fear of painful or damaging treatments administered by distant professionals, being helpless, the demands to fit into the institution, or drug side effects. If you feel anxious or disturbed it might help you to pin this feeling down to causes such as those.

These anxieties are an important and not-well-recognized side effect of conventional medical treatment. Modern medicine, while not treating you as a whole person, creates a good deal of stress while working on a part of you. The bull-in-the-china-shop methods of conventional medicine are nowhere better illustrated than in the efforts it makes to repair the stress it creates. For the usual answer is a tranquillizer and/or a sedative, which leaves the original problem unsolved and adds to it confusion and dullness, as well as the feeling that one is drugged into submission. These drugs may be used more for the benefit of staff than patients, for they quieten down the patient on the outside, never mind the storm still raging within, and relieve the staff of the responsibility of looking after minds as well as bodies.

Stress is a side effect in that it delays recovery.[26] Anxiety makes for more pain and less sleep, reduced appetite and blood flow.[27] It leads to complications after surgery, and more chance of catching infections in hospital.[28] Stresses in medical wards are less than those felt by surgical patients[29] for whom special measures to reduce anxiety are given in Chapter 6. But in all cases anxiety and stress should be, and can be, dealt with.

Good Protection Through Good Connection

You are in the hands of the hospital staff. They can allay your anxieties or leave them to fester, they can make mistakes or get things spot on, they can disturb you and delay your recovery or care for you and hasten it. Nurses are taught that good nursing care should include relieving the anxieties of patients so as to reduce complications during treatment.[30]

One way you can win aid for your fears is to be very clear about your need for information. Many stresses are deflated by the feeling that you are in control, that you decide things along with your doctor and you are given full and honest information so that you can be involved in your treatment. Many studies have shown the benefits of fully preparing patients with information about what they will feel and what will happen, how long they will take to recover and what the procedures are. In one case post-surgical infections were reduced by half when patients were given this kind of preparation.[31]

Staff fail to volunteer information either because they are too busy and tired, or because they feel it wouldn't help you to know. You should insist in your pre-hospital consultation, and in hospital itself:

● That you need full information on all aspects of your treatment.
● That it will aid your recovery and increase your partnership in your treatment.
● That you cannot give your consent without it.
● That you are capable of understanding the information if it is presented to you in common parlance.

● That this should be recorded in your notes so that other staff members and replacements know it.

This is easier than it sounds when you are faced by a brisk preoccupied young nurse, or a curt superior doctor who looks as if he's permanently on his way to resuscitate somebody. So here are some tips on relating to staff.

Don't forget that hospital staff are human too, and may be receiving a daily dose of anxiety, alienation and institutional life for years on end. Nurses may start off as warm independent young girls having to nurse bewildered suffering adults who are scorned if they show any feeling. They have to do what the doctors say, bear the brunt of their failures and receive no credit. Try not to antagonize the nurses. Your doctor should receive your questions and, if necessary, admonishments. Treat the nurses as your allies. That is what they are trained to be even if they are squeezed out of this role by doctors' power.

Talk to the nurses and doctors about themselves. Look them in the eyes. Ask why they are rushed. Find out what they are interested in. It is in your interest to be seen as an individual, as a person.

You want to be seen as a good patient but a questioning and independent one. Be all the things they want you to be – cheerful, friendly, co-operative, considerate – except the grateful victim.

Don't argue, you'll lose. Don't complain, you'll also lose. If you haven't had the information or respect you feel is necessary for your participation in treatment – just drop out. Refuse the medication. The doctor will come and you can tell him the problem on more equal grounds.

Let the doctor know you've done your homework. He'll respect you more. Ask intelligent questions. You will cease to be a number in a bed.

If communication breaks down, use an arbitrator, an intermediary. Your friend, an occupational therapist, or the hospital social worker can be called to your aid.

Prepare the staff as they prepare you. Tell them from the beginning that you are a natural-minded person and against any and all drugs unless they are an absolute and essential part of the treatment. They won't know otherwise. Here is a case which illustrates what can be gained from this kind of approach:

Robert Mason, a 32-year-old cancer patient at the Royal Marsden, told me how he felt it was extremely important to know all about his illness. If he didn't know what was happening he couldn't help himself. He insisted on seeing the X-rays, talking to doctors – and taking and reading his case notes. The staff resented this; they only knew about it when he gave them back. But he persuaded them to support him by saying 'I have created my illness, I take responsibility for it and I know I will get better.' Although they thought him an oddball they were enlisted to prepare his special natural foods, to give him enemas, and to play and sometimes even listen to his relaxation tapes.

Last, bit not least, *trust the staff*. It will help you, and them, to relax. If you have accepted and chosen the treatment, if you have received the information you need, if you are aware of the risks and benefits, relax. You've done all you can; let them do all they can.

Reducing Stress and Aiding Recovery with Relaxation and Imagery

There are well-tried methods of relaxation taught to millions of people to reduce stress and tension which have been rated by researchers as better at this job than tranquillizers.[32] These methods are used to lower blood pressure, control psychomatic problems such as asthma and to improve wellbeing.[33] There is a great deal of evidence of their effectiveness.[34]

Occasionally relaxation methods are taught in local health centres; sadly they are rarely taught in hospitals where they are most needed. The calm and energy that they bring would not only aid in your recovery, but help those who are caring for you. They would help you to rest, sleep and recuperate even if your ward is a bit like Clapham Junction.

There are a very few holistic-minded nurses who understand this. Here is an account by a nurse who tried:

> 'Not long after I arrived I began an evening activity offering relaxation techniques integrating yoga sketches, deep breathing and guided imagery. Patients learned to envision their bodies relaxing and imagine themselves in a peaceful, safe place. They often fell asleep before their customary request for a sleeping pill, and in the morning the patients did not experience their usual medication hangovers.' The nurse, unfortunately, failed to move the doctors. 'My innovations were not appreciated and the reaction seemed to be, "Who does she think she is? After all she is only a nurse." I resigned shortly thereafter.'[35]

Relaxation

The basis of all these methods is relaxation, and this is how it is achieved. First, lie flat and comfortable, if possible without a pillow or with only one. In the case of stomach or back problems it may be more comfortable to bend the knees. At certain times each day, when you know the ward is quiet, and there is likely to be a pause in the endless bustle, you heal yourself. You turn off the light shining in your eyes if you can, and begin to feel the parts of your body. First the toes on the right foot, then the sole and the heel, let them feel heavy, solid, quiet, and relaxed. Then all the other parts of the right leg, then the left, part by part. This way you relax each bit of you from the tip of the toes to the top hair of the head. Now feel the wave of relaxation move through your body and out as you exhale and feel with every breath more deeply relaxed. Enjoy the feeling. You are held up supported and yet light and warm as if floating on water. You are calm and relaxed, calm and relaxed.

Practice this before an unpleasant procedure, before sleep, if there is pain, or at any time. It may be hard to learn relaxation in hospital with all the disturbance (although Professor Jarvis, a world authority on medical stress, used to teach patients to relax using the disturbance – the murmur of voices, the bubble of fluids – with remarkable results).[36] So try and learn it before you go to hospital and bring a tape of progressive relaxation with you.

Once you have learnt to relax properly you can use it as a starting point for various kinds of self-healing methods. You can give yourself affirmations, quiet verbal instructions to your body and mind, of the type recommended by Dr Ainslie Meares and Dr Ian Pearce,[37] such as:

Relax, Relax, Relax,
Completely calm,
At peace, utterly at peace,
Feel this peace spreading through me
In my face, in my body, in my mind and breath,
Breathing easily

Relax, Relax, Relax,
Nature is at rest,
Relaxation renews strength,
Restores strength of mind and body
Strength of body is in calmness of mind

These can be general, or directed to particular organs or parts of the body in brief, energizing 'conversations' with each part.

A variation of this method is autogenic training (AT) which can be learnt before going to hospital. It is an excellent psychological preparation for hospital, designed and taught by aware doctors. AT teaches people to enter and use the state of 'passive concentration' – the deeply relaxed yet aware state we have described – by focusing on sensations of heaviness and warmth in the body. These are the stages:

1. Concentrate on the heaviness of each part of the body, e.g. 'My right arm is heavy'.
2. Concentrate on the warmth in each part of the body, e.g. 'My right arm is warm'.
3. Be aware of the heartbeat and feel its regularity: 'My heartbeat is calm'.
4. Be aware of the calm regularity of the breath, e.g. 'My breathing is calm and regular'.
5. Be aware of warmth in the abdominal area: 'My solar plexus is warm' (omit this exercise if there is an abdominal condition or bleeding from abdominal organs).
6. Be aware of coolness in the forehead: 'My forehead is cool'.
7. Come back to yourself with 'I am refreshed and alert'.

There are further series of affirmations which can be used to heal various parts of the body, which should be taught by an AT instructor a month before entry to hospital.

Imagery
A direction to go in from deep relaxation is to use the state to arouse good feelings in the body. You could imagine yourself being massaged over your whole body with warm oil, giving you a lovely warm feeling. After some time with this imagination you could imagine yourself massaged with light. Or you could imagine yourself on a beach, hearing the sound of the ocean, smelling the fresh breeze and feeling the light and warmth of the sun on your body. Imagine that you are lying in the sand letting it run through your hands and feet.

It is useful to give permission and encouragement to the medical treatment you are receiving. Imagine the drugs spreading through your body and healing you. Imagine also your kidney and liver working to clean them out efficiently after they have done their job. Imagine the circulation cleaning and sweeping all the residues of disease. Think about the images which 'turn you on'. For example if you can get pleasurably lost in an English country garden when you smell real lavender, take a sachet into hospital with you and use it to help the images. After the war in the Lebanon healers were working in hospitals in the North of Israel with wounded soldiers. Each soldier received packages of pure aromatic herbs. One gravely wounded soldier would sniff it each time the pain became unbearable and cry out 'Hotel De Luxe'!

Imagery is a powerful process. One young man came out of surgery after an injury in a terrible state. He was screaming with pain, shocked and scared. He couldn't sleep for days because he was sure that he would die in his sleep. His sister, who was an expert in the use of imagery, was called in. She quietly suggested that he walk in his garden. He calmed down. She suggested to him that he give the body two hours' rest. The next day when she came he was angry. He had slept, but why only two hours? She worked with images to clean his body and his psyche of the memories of the injury and the surgery. Gradually she taught him to use images himself, and he was soon rapidly getting better.

You can work on images yourself, but it is always better to have some help in inducing the right image for you and your condition. One patient may be able to concentrate easily and precisely on a part of the body, and this can achieve results without particular affirmations or messages of encouragement. Another person might respond to a more general image of the 'walking by the sea' type. For example a 65-year-old man was in hospital because an operation wound to pin broken bones in his foot had become seriously infected. Blood supply was poor and he was in danger of amputation. A therapist who worked with imagery was called by the family. She simply asked him to visit the area. What does he see there in his mind's eye? He began to carefully examine the area in his imagination. He saw the wound and saw it full of blood. As soon as this patient felt himself, the panic left and healing returned. By concentrating very well on this specific area in a concrete way there was a response. He was walking in a few days.

Find a therapist – a psychotherapist, nurse or counsellor – who is conversant with imagery. Obtain some training in the use of relaxation and imagery. Try and make tapes when you are strong to help you enter the state of passive concentration when you are weak.

Make use of paramedics who are sometimes trained in these techniques. Occupational therapists often teach relaxation to patients suffering from respiratory problems. They also use techniques such as reminiscence therapy with confused or aged patients. This involves encouraging patients to remember experiences and even tastes of their past. It is not far away from imagery work. They are also responsible for dealing with side effects of long-term hospital stays and can act as informal counsellors.

Therapists in Hospital

Physiotherapists, occupational therapists, dietitians, art and music therapists and social workers all work within the NHS hospital system. They are a unique resource for the surviving patient, particularly if they have learnt special complementary methods to aid comfort and recovery, such as breathing, relaxation, massage, acupuncture or counselling. Normally these therapists are ordered by the doctor, for example to help with breathing and mobility after an operation. They in turn can often report back to the doctor on your behalf, say in the case of an unwelcome drowsiness from drug side effects.

If you hear from the medical staff that a paramedic has a skill you feel would be valuable for you, or you want to speak to one, ask the sister (they are not the formidable starched white battleships they used to be). Patients are not entitled to refer themselves but your request will normally result in the paramedic popping in to see you. After that it's up to you. This is often the easiest way to obtain complementary treatment in hospital.

You can sometimes find one or other complementary therapy practised by a doctor or a nurse in the hospital, and you could ask your doctor to arrange that such a person sees you. However, this ought to be arranged with your consultant before you enter hospital – you are less likely to be able to organize it once in the ward.

Furthermore you should meet with that staff member beforehand in case they are not suitable. For example you may hear there is an acupuncturist in hospital and you are admitted assuming you can ask to see him for insomnia or drug side effects. However, like many medical acupuncturists, it may turn out that he only knows about pain and may not even admit the possibility that acupuncture can be useful for anything else.

Complementary therapists such as homeopaths, acupuncturists, reflexologists, healers etc. can come and visit you from the outside but you should ask permission of your consultant or doctor, preferably before admission. You should explain why you need the therapist in such a way that the consultant will understand. Don't say 'for my aura', as he'll reply 'oral what?', say it's for anxiety, psychological support, or pain relief without drugs which you are sensitive to. If he thinks it will help you recover more quickly there is a 90% chance that he will not object. After all he will get the credit for your successful recovery! Even a government-issued brochure on patients' rights mentions that spiritual healers can visit patients in hospital.[13] He may not be very happy about the idea though, and you can expect a token resistance. It will be much easier if the complementary therapist you wish to bring in is medically qualified.

Where you expect or receive complete refusal to have a complementary medical visit, which happens in some 10% of cases, you can usually disguise a healer, reflexologist, or hypnotist as a close friend or counsellor and get away with a surreptitious treatment.

Yoga During Prolonged Bed-rest

If you are set for a long period in bed there are certain consequences which you should be aware of. Immobility causes wasting of muscles, leakage of minerals from the bones and the possibility of blood clots or sluggish circulation. It becomes more difficult to get rid of toxins due to drugs and digestion. All the pumps, vessels, and valves in the body slow down.

Yoga is the best self-care method under these conditions. The word 'yoga' may conjure up visions of patients doing headstands on their beds all along the ward. But it has subtler aspects. Stretching followed by deeply relaxing is an excellent exercise which can be carried out in bed, provided that new operation scars are not stretched. As you stretch imagine you are tall and long, and stretch one side and the other, and each of your limbs in turn. You can rotate the joints of arms, legs, and neck, describing circles with the feet and hands. Tensing and relaxing individual muscle groups throughout the body, including the perineal region (the crotch), is very helpful in getting the circulation going, lifting mood, muscle tone and general wellbeing. If you are sitting you can add twists of the trunk and sideways bending and swaying. You can do shoulder lifts, and describe circles with your arms. Many yoga teachers will be able to teach you relevant postures.

However, breathing methods are the main gift of yoga to the sick or recovering. Steady, paced breathing in the yoga fashion is one of the best of all methods for calming the mind and reducing tension and anxiety, and it acts fast. Hormonal changes indicating a reduction in stress occur within a couple of minutes of starting yoga breathing. The extra ventilation and oxygenation of the blood gives energy, drives out accumulated toxins and drug hangovers and can lift depression.[38] Physiotherapists teach deep breathing after operations to help start up sluggish anaesthetized organs and prevent lung problems. But all patients in hospital would benefit, and you don't need the physiotherapist.

In case you cannot quite see the connection between your breath and the rest of the problems besetting your poor frame during medical treatment, let me point out three facts. First, deep breathing brings more oxygen to the parts that need it most while under stress: your brain for example. Second, it is known to shift automatic nervous activity in the body from the alarm type to the alarm-over type. Third, one of the waste products of our metabolism is a substance called lactate, which builds up and causes tiredness during physical exercise. High levels of lactate can induce panic and anxiety and they are reduced by breathing. A recent study at St. Bartholomews Hospital in London has demonstrated clearly that breathing from the diaphragm cuts out panic.

In a survey of cancer patients who used yoga, carried out by Dr Robin Monro in Cambridge, half said that yoga helped them to avoid tranquillizers and other pills, half said it helped avoid pain, while all of them stated that they had a more positive attitude to their disease and treatment. 'The cleansing breath on recovery immediately after the head operation expelled the anaesthetic', wrote one woman. 'Then, alternative nostril breathing helped to balance my emotions and induced sleep.'[39]

There are two types of yoga breathing to consider, one more calming and one more energizing. The principles of the calming breath are regularity and an exhalation which is steady, controlled, and twice as long as the inhalation:

● Take a long even breath down to the stomach.
● Hold it for 1½ times as long.
● Exhale steadily, controlling the passage of the breath by restricting it in the throat, for twice as long as the inhalation.
● Try it with both nostrils at once, then each in turn.
● Concentrate on the feeling of the breath going in, the suspension when you retain it, and the release and outflow.

The other breathing technique is diaphragmatic breathing:

● Take a steady breath that is drawn in more by the expansion of the belly than by the chest.
● Feel the breath filling the body right down to the belly like water filling a bottle.
● Exhale by contracting the belly and feel the emptying process.

Debility Diets and Recovery Foods

' "Well then, can I do anything to reinforce my defences? What about food, for instance, should I follow a special diet?"
The doctor shook his head. "Diet has nothing to do with cancer." He said "Just make sure that you eat plenty of good nourishing food to build up your strength. That's all."
"Do you realize how abysmal the food is in this hospital?"
"Oh, I've seen worse. And you won't be here all that long." '
The response one cancer patient received to her question[40] seems to sum up accurately the official position on hospital food: you'll survive it. But will you? Half of the patients in some general wards in the US suffer from protein-calorie malnutrition, and patients hospitalized for more than two weeks tend to become run down because of poor food,[41] a situation that even the British Medical

Journal has complained about[42]. In one of the premium hospitals in the country, one quarter of the patients were found to be under-nourished, and many had less iron and vitamins than the international recommendations for the healthy, let alone the sick[43] Some hospital meals are so impoverished that you would have to eat two of them each time just to get the minimum requirements of minerals such as magnesium and zinc,[44] and vitamins such as C and D.[45,46]

The lack of vitamins particularly affects the elderly in hospitals because apart from the poor diet, they don't absorb vitamins properly. One study found that half the elderly in medical care had vitamin C levels in their white blood cells which were as low as those of people suffering from scurvy.[47] Yet it is known that even small deficiencies of vitamin C in white blood cells inhibit their immune checking of the body, and the repairing of wounds, and over 10 years ago the British Medical Journal was advising all hospitals to give vitamin C supplements to the elderly.[48]

The elderly in care also suffer from chronic low levels of the B vitamins: 'It's a sub-clinical vitamin deficiency. That means that there are no clinical signs. But it's very debilitating because it doesn't permit them to feel well, concentrate, or function properly, and it has a dire effect on their ability to resist disease and infection.' This is how Professor Herman Baker of the New Jersey Medical School described it.[44]

While your hospital diet gives you less than a healthy person, your needs are much greater. Drugs destroy vitamins, stress uses them up, and antibiotics can prevent them being absorbed in the diet. At the same time larger quantities of vitamins such as vitamin C, and minerals such as zinc, are needed to ensure proper healing of surgical wounds[49] and to protect you from infections and complications.[50] A study of 500 patients in New Jersey hospitals showed that those with low blood protein from poor diet were four times more likely to have complications.

There are several reasons for such poor nutrition, the main one being that medical staff are uninterested in the question of *optimum* (as opposed to minimum) nutrition. So hospitals do not employ nutritionists to oversee their food, and they never monitor your food consumption and relate it to your individual requirements. The other problem is that of institutional catering. The meals have to be prepared in large quantities at low cost. So out go choice, taste and balance. In come processed, refined, dehydrated and frozen foods. Hospitals have missed a golden opportunity to give a residential course to the sick on nutrition and health. Instead they often do not keep to the public guidelines suggested by the Health Education Council.

The kind of food received by one cancer patient on arrival at a

London hospital was 'Thin tinned soup, thin leathery meat, drowned vegetables, sliced white bread, tinned "plastic" fruit compote, the kind of detestable food that left one both bloated and hungry . . . food that smacked of a third rate seaside café.'[40] There can be little doubt that such food inhibits your recovery and is a significant side effect of a hospital stay. Fortunately it is one that you can easily rectify.

The Food You Need in Hospital

A hospital is the very place where you should have the best meals of your life. The food should be highly nutritious with plenty of protein for healing and recovery. The keys to healthy eating in hospital can be summed up by four don'ts:

No empty calories. That is, no food whatsoever that is refined in such a way as to remove its extra fibres, vitamins, minerals, colours and natural plant constituents. This is especially important if you only eat small amounts. Thus white flour, instant mashed potato, refined cooking oil, sugar, custard powder, are all empty, while wholewheat flour, whole vegetables, unrefined or cold-pressed oils and molasses, are the corresponding whole foods. Professor Bender calculated, in his British Medical Journal editorial on hospital food, that patients can be forced to obtain all their essential vitamins and minerals from one third of their diet.[42] The rest is just empty calories. Stodge is the old-fashioned word.

No tinned, overcooked or preserved foods. Get hold of a fresh apple, don't have the tinned stewed apple. Get fresh peas, don't have those things that seemed to have been peas. They too have been emptied of nutrients by preserving and overcooking.

No ancient relics. A lettuce should taste like one and be fresh, otherwise the salad, which may be your main meal, will not be worth eating. It will fill you up and give you little. Ideally food should be grown organically and brought straight to you. An orange can lose 80% of its vitamin C on storage, and chemically grown food has less nutrients than organically grown food. For example garlic can have ten times more of the medicinally active component, allicin, if it is grown in live compost rather than sterilized soil.

No chemical cocktails. You cannot taste the preservatives, additives, colouring and flavouring agents, but you can probably guess that the bright red jelly in front of you has never seen a real strawberry. Mass catered hospital food tends to have a lot of these additives, even though two London hospitals have shown that they can discharge some young patients just by feeding them additive-free foods.[51]

Instead seek natural, wholesome unprocessed foods for example:

● Protein foods: soya, lentils, sesame, chickpeas, free-range eggs, cheese, fish, organ meats, tahini.
● Carbohydrate foods: porridge oats, wholewheat (not just 'brown') bread, root vegetables (esp. sweet potatoes), brown rice, millet or buckwheat.
● Fibre/vitamin foods: salads, fresh fruit, dark green and yellow vegetables.
● Fats: cheese, cold-pressed oils, tahini, avocado, nuts, seeds.

One of the best recovery diets you can find is macrobiotic. This involves a fine balance of food factors which can be designed according to your particular condition. Based on traditional Japanese methods of cooking for the spirit as well as the stomach, it concentrates on vegetables, brown rice, bean products and sea products. If you are in hospital, try and get advice on a natural diet specially for you from a naturopath or macrobiotic instructor. Whoever can prepare the food for you should join in.

Recovery Foods
If you want to obtain some good concentrated nutritious foods, or natural liquid foods for a patient who is not eating, here are some suggestions:

Miso soup. The doyen of macrobiotic cooking, made from miso (fermented soya bean paste), spring onions and dried vegetables, and sometimes brown rice paste. There is nothing better. It is what I have after any illness.

Chicken soup. The main thing linking Jews and Chinese is a great respect for chicken soup. If you can get hold of the Chinese version from Chinese or Japanese shops it can contain Royal Jelly or Chinese tonic herbs. It is a powerful restorative but should have bones cooked in it in the traditional way.

Fresh vegetable and fruit juices. Get a friend with a juicer to keep a relay of fresh juices arriving at your bedside. Green vegetables, onions and carrots contain most of the vitamins you need. Juicing extracts them without the destructive process of cooking. Juices are very important to those on restrictive or liquid diets, and people who do not have a good appetite. They are tasty and contain many vitamins. They are by no means the same as canned, bottled or boxed juices to which they bear the same relation as trees to paper.

Tofu, or bean curd. This is concentrated coagulated soya bean extract.

It is easy to digest, pure, full of protein, and can easily be combined with other dishes.

Onions and garlic. These are key vegetables on the recovery menu. They are full of unusual minerals and vitamins. They help in detoxification of drugs and chemicals, stimulating the liver and urinary system. They act against saturated fats and most important of all, they are powerful anti-infectives and will protect the body against infections and clear up any that arrive.[52] Garlic is almost as powerful as many antibiotics and a lot safer – but see page 148 about how to take it.

Natural live yoghurt (see page 65) made from goats' milk is especially good.

The Water
You may not eat and drink a great deal in hospital. What you do take in should be impeccable. Water from the tap is not. As with much of the food you meet in hospitals and other institutions, it doesn't contain all the things you need and does contain some you don't. For example fluorine in tap water can delay healing of bones and tissues, according to one study,[53] especially if it is combined with fluorine in toothpaste and fluorine compounds (of which many pesticides are composed) contaminating foods.

Obtain bottled mineral or spring water. Make sure it gives the source on the label. A confidential survey of bottled water in the US found that 21 of 50 companies obtained their water from the tap. Mineral water is widely used on the Continent and in the USSR as a specific treatment of various conditions such as arthritis, hepatitis, gastritis and bronchitis, each one requiring water of a different composition. A good mineral water can give you extra calcium and magnesium, selenium and iron.

How to Get the Right Foods
It is all very well knowing what foods to get. But how do you get it? The first step is to request natural food from the hospital. You may be lucky. Some hospitals offer concessions towards wholefoods. A few hospitals in the UK offer brown rice as a choice, because of the extra B vitamins and fibre it contains. University College Hospital gives wholemeal bread or high-fibre white (choose the former). Another hospital has a natural foods counter – for staff only! But it's a start. It would be best to write to the administrator beforehand mentioning any special diets such as vegetarianism and stating that you are used to natural unprocessed additive-free foods. Say you are sensitive to food additives. Ask what arrangements can be made to

accommodate you. Then when you get your first meal, if it comes out of a tin ask the sister if you can see the dietitian.

The dietitian is in a position to help you. Dietitians have to be referred by doctors, but your request will probably be answered anyway. The dietitian, at last, will be someone who knows about the food. Her or his job is to design diets for special cases: light but nutritious meals for people without appetite because of their drug treatment, or frequent small or liquid meals, with special nutrient-formula drinks for people after stomach surgery for example. You should ask the dietitian first about the hospital food – how fresh it is, whether the vitamins like B, E, C, and minerals like iron and zinc, are sufficient, and how many additives and preservatives it contains. This will help you to assess the meals. Then ask her if there are any special vitamin requirements because of the drugs you are taking. Then discuss with her your wish for nutritious natural wholefoods.

Now the dietitian is used to persuading patients, who are in hospital because of a lifelong diet of jam butties and fish and chips, to eat some salads. You will be putting the shoe on the other foot. She may agree with you and complain that the medical staff don't care about nutrition and the kitchens get no money and the patients wouldn't want natural food anyway. Or she may be unsympathetic, reprimanding you for believing magazine articles and championing the hospital food by vague generalizations about its nutritiousness. In either case she will be able to arrange with the kitchen to give you a special diet, or at least a salad at the expense of the pudding. Cancer patients at University College Hospital and the Royal Marsden have been helped by dietitians to receive vegetable juices and a special natural diet. One UCH hospital dietitian I spoke to went on the strict diet recommended by the British Cancer Help Centre herself for two weeks to see what it is like, and tries to coordinate it herself within the hospital. Some surprises do occasionally turn up. One day complete macrobiotic Japanese-style food became available in one Philadelphia hospital along with the traditional packaged fare. It turned out that a surgeon at this hospital had had cancer and was in despair at the possible treatment options available. Driving along the freeway in his gloom, he picked up a hitchhiker. It turned out that the hitchhiker was a macrobiotic food instructor in a health centre who convinced him of the value of diet where many others had failed. The surgeon got better through the diet, became an enthusiast and established the kitchen.

In average hospitals, however, you can assume that you will have to refuse a good deal of the food and get your companions and friends to run a shuttle. At present about 10% of patient calories are brought in by visitors. If you want to eat wholesome natural food this will have to go up to at least 50%. Home cooking has, of course, the advantage that you get what you want. One patient treated with chemotherapeutic drugs couldn't eat anything the hospital brought her, and she grew weaker. Her daughter discovered the one thing she could take: fruit salad. She brought it four times a day subtly laced with wheatgerm, walnuts, sunflower seeds and sesame seeds, with soya milk poured on top. This was her diet – and in the circumstances it was excellent.

In India, the families of hospital patients see it as their main duty to bring home-cooked food in little caddies. India is a culture where the health-promoting aspects of food are very well understood. It is quite clear that each person has a requirement for particular foods according to his state of health and his constitution. Therefore only the family, who know him, can be relied upon to design recovery diets. The same thing applies in the Far East. According to Janet Marshall all the wards in her Japanese hospital have little kitchens especially for visitors to prepare the food they bring for patients.

Nutritional Assessment

If you are in for long-term hospital or medical institutional care you can ask for a nutritional assessment. A blood test can detect vitamin deficiencies before any obvious symptoms or infections develop. Ask the physician in charge to arrange it. In the UK he may not even know what you are talking about. You can only reply to him that senior staff in a number of major medical centres in the USA recommend it, and you wish to do it privately. Nutritional organizations described in the appendix can arrange it.

Looking After Your Digestion

Drugs (especially antibiotics), immobility, surgery and a change of diet can play havoc with your digestion. Intestinal movement slows down, appetite is lost, nausea, gas, indigestion and constipation are common in hospital leading to more drugs. Quite drastic changes happen to the intestinal population of bacteria. They become invaded by unfriendly species.[54] These species create irritations and food allergies, and they can lead to depression, headache, lethargy, slow recovery[55] and infections after surgery.[56]

The regular bacteria (the bifidobacteria) create certain acids which stimulate the movement of the intestines, and thus get rid of bacterial and toxic wastes from the body.[54] These acids create the right environment for digestion and prevent invasion by strangers. The local bacteria also increase absorbtion of minerals such as calcium, magnesium and potassium, and they make essential vitamins including B_{12}, pantothenic acid and biotin.[57] If antibiotics destroy natural bacteria, the strangers can multiply, creating the symptoms described.

The natural bacteria are encouraged by vegetable fibre in the diet and discouraged by meat products and saturated fats.[58] The vegetable fibre should come from salads and fruit rather than wheat bran which is concentrated and may be an irritant.

Yoghurt contains necessary acids and will help to preserve the natural population against a drug-induced holocaust.[59] Try to have live yoghurt even in smallish amounts three times a day, (unless you are on MAO inhibiting types of antidepressant drugs).

If your digestion is affected by antibiotics and dietary change, instead of laxatives, antacids and so on, take tablets of *Lactobacillus acidophilus*. This helps to repopulate the intestine with the beneficial bacteria. There is evidence that taking acidophilus increases general immunity and prevents infections, adds to vitamin production, and improves general health.[60] Curiously, farmers have long known that they can improve the growth and health of domestic animals by giving Lactobacillus.[61] Such husbandry would be welcome in hospitals.

Massage and Essential Oils to Bring Life and Energy

All through Eastern countries – travelling on Indian trains, in the Thai markets, in a multitude of Japanese clinics, you will see massage. Mothers to children, husbands and wives to each other and children among themselves. I once sat opposite an elderly woman on a train from Calcutta to Benares, who didn't stop rythmically massaging her scalp for the entire day's journey. And you will find as much massage in hospitals as you will in massage parlours.

Massage is more than a pleasure to a hospital patient in bed. It can make a great deal of difference to the way the lymph removes toxic wastes, the way the blood circulates, the movement of inert organs and passageways in the body slowed by drugs, and of course immobile limbs with their tension, cramp and muscle weakness.[62]

Massage for removing wastes and achieving these physiological results should be carried out by a trained masseur. One powerful technique that can be used is *shiatzu*, or Japanese pressure-point massage. This involves prolonged pressure on acupuncture points around the body. It can achieve the relief of specific symptoms as well as to generally awaken and tone up body systems, and keep body and soul together (this is not as flippant as it sounds, for in long-term institutions the 'soul', 'spirit' or 'life-energy' seems to just pack up and go, leading to lifelessness, lethargy and inertia).

Used therapeutically, for example, you can reduce anxiety through pressure on the 'Godly serenity' point at the top of the calf, stimulate the appetite using the 'An-min' point on the outside of the top joint of the little finger, stimulate the circulation on the opposite side of the little finger at the 'El-mu' point, and treat constipation and diahorrea, headache, insomnia, tiredness, pain, or nausea, all symptoms that may crop up as a result of lying in hospital beds under drug treatment. However you need to learn the skill for yourself or ask for a skilled shiatzu practitioner. It cannot be learnt from books.

This does not mean that you cannot massage yourself. Massage of the head and extremities is valuable when you are in bed, at the least because it keeps you active and in touch with yourself. It gives you energy and confidence. Here are a few tips:

● Massage the soles of your feet with your thumbs in a rythmic way, with deep pressure and rotation, especially along the midline and the arch.
● Do the same on the palms of the hands and the base of the fingers.
● A fatigue point is on the middle of the top joint of the little finger and at the top of the nape of the neck: use rhythmic pressure.
● Pain points are on the ankles below and behind the ankle bone and in the joint between thumb and forefinger: use rhythmic pressure.
● Help insomnia by firm stroking of the neck muscles and the lobe of the ear.
● Massage your limbs slowly with long firm strokes, with concentration, for an hour a day.

Essential oils are powerful concentrates of herbs and can be used with massage, or you can just smell them. Most can be taken internally too, at no more than two drops four times a day. Here is a table of suitable oils and their uses:

Oil	Function
Rosemary or Ambergris	Restores circulation to tissues. Relaxes tense muscles. Useful for early bedsores
Basil	Lifts mood and awakens
Balm	Helpful for insomnia
Catnip	Helpful for insomnia
Comfrey	Helps healing, soothes irritations and bedsores
Wheat Germ	Massage over scars, irritations
Lavender	Antiseptic and cleansing oil
Cinnamon and Clove	Warms the limbs
Peppermint	Aids digestion and loosens tension

Note: Don't put oil into the eyes or orifices where it could burn, and check with small quantities first in case of a rare allergic skin reaction. Certain essential oils are not safe to take internally.

Vitamin Supplements: What To Take With You

After all that has been said about food, why should anyone need to take vitamins? The main reason is that extra vitamins are your insurance in case, despite strenuous nutritional efforts, your diet doesn't prove sufficient. Besides, certain vitamins have therapeutic effects in doses much too large to get in the modern diet. There are many reasons why vitamin supplementation is recommended to all hospital patients.

Vitamins help to detoxify the body and clean it of drug residues, anaesthetics, or wastes from poor digestion. They do this either by activating the liver and metabolism (the B vitamins) or by inactivating and burning up poisons directly (e.g. vitamin E, selenium and vitamin C). This is discussed in the drugs chapters.

Vitamins have psychological effects, not as drugs, more as nutrients. Sluggish metabolism, low blood sugar or lack of certain nutrients can produce sleeplessness, fatigue and irritability. Minerals and B vitamins counteract this.[63] Premature senility and confusion which is so common among the elderly in hospital has been linked with poor diets and partially reversed by thiamine.[64] Certain amino acids such as tyrosine and tryptophan, which are normally part of the diet, can reduce pain, induce sleep and reduce depression when they are taken as concentrated supplements.[65]

Vitamins and minerals can make a dramatic difference in the capacities of the immune system. Quite small deficiencies in zinc, for example, can inhibit the function of the thymus gland, which pours out cells that defend the body against infections. There is also a special need for extra vitamins A and C, when your resistance is low and there are plenty of opportunities of infection.

Vitamins enhance wound healing and surgical recovery, especially vitamins C, E, pantothenic acid and vitamin B_6.

Vitamins increase absorbtion, digestion and metabolism of food. If you are only eating small amounts, vitamin supplements are essential to make full use of what you do eat. For example extra vitamin C can increase absorbtion of iron by several times.

Vitamins and minerals can prevent damage from insufficient movement and sunlight. Lack of exercise leaches calcium from the bones and they become weaker. Lack of sunlight reduces vitamin D levels, as do antacids, barbiturates, laxatives and other drugs. Vitamin D and magnesium control the amount of calcium laid down

Nutritional Supplementation in Hospital

Food Factor	FDA Standard Recommendation for Adults	Recommended Average Hospital Supplementation	Usual Sources
B vitamins:			
B_1	1·5 mg	10 mg	wheat germ, molasses, yeast, liver, unpolished rice
B_2	1·7 mg	10 mg	
*B_3	20 mg	100 mg	
*B_6	2·2 mg	20 mg	
B_{12}	0·006 mg	0·006 mg	
biotin	0·3 mg	0·6 mg	
*pantothenate	10 mg	100 mg	
Vitamin A	5000 IU	20,000 IU	As for Vit. D + carrots and yellow vegetables
*Vitamin C with bioflavonoids	60 mg	2 gm	fresh fruit
Vitamin D	400 IU	1000 IU	fish, egg yolk, cod liver oil, sunshine
*Vitamin E	15 IU	300 IU	leafy vegetables, wheat germ, cold-pressed oils
Minerals:			
calcium	800 mg	2 gm	seafood, cheese, yoghurt
magnesium	350 mg	600 mg	seafood, nuts and vegetables
iron	10 mg	20 mg	meat, especially liver, dark green vegetables, molasses or supplement
zinc	15 mg	25 mg	seafood, liver, yeast

Note: This is an average guide. A nutritionally oriented holistic physician, nurse or adviser should be able to design a diet and supplement for you. The above dosages represent modest use of vitamins therapeutically. Larger doses can be useful but should be supervised.

IU is *International Units*, an agreed convention to describe doses of certain vitamins.

* These should be obtained from supplements as it is hard to obtain them from the diet in sufficient quantities.

in the bones, and the absorbtion of calcium.[66] In a study at an old-age home in Boston, during the winter the lack of sun reduced the amount of calcium absorbed to one quarter of the amount ingested. Lack of calcium leads to weak bones, weak muscles, tension and raised pain sensitivity. The vitamins involved are Vitamin D, calcium and magnesium, which should be taken if you are in bed for some weeks.

Further evidence for these assertions is presented in the various chapters later in the book. At this point we will develop a standard list of vitamins which you might consider taking with you into hospital to cover all eventualities. For further details, see reference 67.

Herbal Remedies for Bedsores and Other Problems

Herbs and natural remedies are *your* medicines, they are available for you to find, try, prepare and use, and they can be your answer to a range of distressing problems that may crop up. We will concentrate here only on problems that arise from the stay in the hospital itself, insofar as they are unnecessary side effects of the treatment you are receiving.

Bedsores

These are as a result of lack of movement, pressure, and lack of circulation in the peripheral areas of the body. They are *not* an inescapable part of long stays in hospital, as they can be prevented by excellent nursing, some physiotherapy and exercise, and a balanced nutritious high-protein diet.

If you are at risk of developing bedsores, or have them already, it is doubly important that you take vitamin supplements. Bedsores respond well to vitamin E, which brings oxygen to the periphery of the body. This is the most important vitamin but B vitamins help to utilize the high-protein diet that is part of treatment. Make sure you do not take any saturated or refined fats and oils, which inhibit oxygenation. Take instead cold-pressed wheat germ, sunflower, soya or corn oils. If this is impossible buy capsules of GLA, Gamma Linoleic Acid, and take them regularly.

Several local applications have been successfully used to stop bedsores. The first is aloe vera gel. It helps to keep the skin moist and soft, and has powerful anti-infective and anti-inflammatory actions. You can buy it as a lotion or salve and rub it on. The second is vitamin E enriched wheat germ oil. This can be bought in capsules which should be pierced and spread. It is more effective when bedsores are not yet well established. A third treatment is rosemary oil, in some kind of base. This too is better at prevention than cure. It also encourages circulation in the periphery and like vitamin E, is an anti-oxidant. Try these preparations three or four times a day.

Classical herbal remedies for treating bedsores are astringents such as witch hazel, mucilaginous agents which moisten and stimulate new skin growth, such as comfrey root extract and certain seaweeds, and agents to help microcirculation, including arnica and rosemary. These agents can be found ready made up; or obtain a herbalist's prescription. They are far more effective external preparations than anything available within conventional medicine, which treats bedsores with zinc oxide and barrier creams. The herbal preparations can always be rubbed in before the barrier creams.

Sleeplessness

Sleep is the best thing you can do with your time in hospital. Most healing happens then, for the hormones shift their emphasis from waking nervous awareness to the mending and house-cleaning of the body when we sleep.[68] Sleeplessness can have external reasons such as noise, and all you can do about that is bring earplugs in your hospital kit. Internally there are several ways of dealing with it.

First, don't take sedatives. They have side effects, they impose an extra stress on the liver, steal nutrients, prevent self-care and inhibit recovery. Breathing and exercises in hospital (see above) are the best methods, combined with a sanguine attitude to the lack of sleep. It probably is a natural response to disturbances, upset rhythms, or a lack of fresh air and exercise.

Take a strong chamomile tea before you go to bed. In one study patients were given a strong chamomile tea before heart catheterisation. Several actually fell asleep during what is usually an uncomfortable procedure. A holistic nurse described how she started making chamomile tea at bedtime in her ward of depressed insomniac women. She began to give chamomile tea in the evenings instead of the usual sedatives. She described how many of the women slept without a sedative for the first time in years, and how several of them woke up in the morning fresh rather than crushed by a drug hangover. Unfortunately she was stopped by doctors who said that the chamomile tea might interfere with some experimental drugs they were using, which she found quite incredible.[35]

If chamomile tea does not work there is still something stronger and yet much safer than sedatives – this is valerian root. In contrast to chamomile tea it cannot usually be bought in tea bags although you may find it as part of night-time herbal mixtures. Your companion can always bring a flask in the evening. Incidentally, never have coffee, tea, or Coca-Cola within four hours of bedtime.

Herb teas are a much healthier replacement.

Tryptophan is an amino acid that can be taken before bedtime as a safe effective natural sedative. It is available on prescription in the UK. In America obtain it from holistic practitioners. It has been successfully tried in hospital.[69]

Organic problems

Indigestion, heartburn and gas occur because of drugs, anaesthetics, change of diet, stomach infections and tension. Antacids do not work very well, stop absorbtion of valuable nutrients and can give you side effects of tiredness and poor digestion. Instead take slippery elm, marshmallow root, or comfrey root as teas. They are soothing and at the same time promote healing in all the tissues. Peppermint tea relieves cramp and nausea and peppermint oil even relieves irritable bowel syndrome.[70]

For gas you can use garlic, together with charcoal tablets, an old-time remedy that works. But aromatic spices, particularly cinnamon and ginger, are a very good way of relieving gas and settling the stomach, particularly because they are warming, benefiting the circulation, and also anti-infective in case of stomach infection. They help absorbtion of food and medicines. You can add these aromatics to any hot drink at ⅓ – ¼ teaspoonful a time.

Constipation is a common hospital problem. It can be dealt with partly by a diet with a great deal of roughage of different kinds, especially vegetables, salads and fresh fruit. Instead of conventional laxatives use the soothing herbs mentioned in the previous section, and if necessary, use a teaspoonful of ispaghula husk (plantago seed) or commercial laxative herb mixtures.

Headaches arise from constipation, from toxins in the blood that haven't cleared, from stuffy atmosphere and positive charged ions, from tension and stress and a variety of other causes. You should refuse strong cheeses or cocoa if you have recurrent headaches in hospital and use tiger balm, or oils of mint, eucalyptus and cajuput or rosemary, rubbing them into the temples, and massaging the nape of the neck. Herb teas or tablets consisting of echinacea and St Johns Wort (Hypericum) are effective blood purifiers and can relieve headaches resulting from accumulated waste products in the blood. Juniper is a natural way of increasing the washing out of these toxins from the blood.

Tiredness and Lethargy

The best herbs to take if you are tired from the cumulative

effects of illness and treatment are oriental restoratives. The most famous is ginseng, and it has been well tried for this purpose. Ginseng used to be more of a myth than a medicine; now it is a mixture of the two. The Chinese have a deep understanding of those in between states of health which are neither illness nor wellness. Their ancient medical system puts great store on preventive measures, and herbal or acupuncture treatment in this in between state can halt susceptibilities, diseases and disabilities. Ginseng is one of the best remedies to be discovered as a true preventative and restorative medicine. It is used to increase energy and alertness during chronic illness, recovery, weakness and old age. It is known to act on the hormonal circuitry of the body to prevent the harmful effects of stress, and to adjust the physiology – including blood sugar, blood pressure, the metabolism and body temperature.[71] Its use against exhaustion has been supported by a great many scientific studies[72,73] and applied in practice. It is successfully used by Asian and Soviet sportsmen, divers, soldiers and cosmonauts to adjust their bodies to extremes.

The use of ginseng during recovery has a modern tradition in addition to its ancient one. In Soviet hospitals and in the Far East ginseng or its relatives are used to give strength to recovering patients and prevent complications. In one study of 120 patients who underwent serious abdominal or gynaecological surgery, half were given the active ingredients of ginseng, and half a placebo. Those treated with ginseng had better liver function, put on weight faster and felt better.[73] Similar studies have been carried out in the USSR with a related herb, eleutherococcus.[74]

Ginseng is an ideal recovery herb and should be in the tray of remedies your nurse brings round. It would save a lot of NHS money. However since you have to buy it, and it is expensive, here are some rules: buy whole roots or root pieces; if not available buy thick paste extract or ground root. Never buy tea or liquid extract. Choose Asian rather than European brands. Asian red ginseng is better than white and well worth the extra money, but it must be a Korean or Chinese product. You should start taking ginsing in the recovery phase, not the acute phase, of an illness, at a dose of 1 gm a day minimum. Eleutherococcus is a cheaper but less effective alternative.

REFERENCES

1. **Stockwell, F.** *The Unpopular Patient*, London, Royal College of Nursing (1972).

2. Geiger, J. in: Howard J. and Strauss, J. (eds) *Humanising Health Care*, N.Y. John Wiley (1975).
3. Feder, G. *Brit. Med. J.*, **290** 322 (1985).
4. Davidson, J. J. *Alt. Medicine*, 7–8 (February 1985).
5. Falk, S. A. and Woods, N. F. *New Eng. J. Med.* 774–781 (11 October 1973).
6. Shapiro, R. A. and Berland, T. *New Eng. J. Med.* 1236–1239 (14 December 1972)
7. Douek, E. *et al. The Lancet*, **2** 1110-3 (1976).
8. Inlander, C. B., Weiner, E. *Take This Book to Hospital with You*, People's Medical Society, Rodale Press. Pa. (1985).
9. Editorial, *Postgraduate Medicine*, January (1980).
10. Fulder, S. J. *The Handbook of Complementary Medicine*, Coronet, London (1987).
11. Bennett, G. *Patients and Their Doctors*.
12. The College of Health, London (see appendix for address) publishes lists of waiting times at UK hospitals.
13. National Consumer Council, *Patients' Rights*, HMSO (1983).
14. Baile, W. F. *et al, J. Behav. Med.* **2** 85 (1979).
15. Editorial *Brit. Med. J.* **289** 1709–1712 (1984).
16. Thibault, G. E. *et al, New Engl. J. Med.* **302** 938-942 (1980).
17. Estola, T. *et al, J. Hyg. Camb.*, **83** 59 (1979).
18. David, T. *et al, Am. J. Phys. Med.*, **39** 111-3 (1950).
19. Martin, S. J. *Alt. Med.*, 17 (March 1984).
20. Information given informally by National Public Health Laboratory, Division of Hospital Infection, Colindale, London NW9.
21. Hartsfield, J. and Clopton J. R. *Soc. Sci. and Medicine,* **5** 529-533 (1985).
22. Clark A. J. and Affonso, D. *Child Bearing, A Nursing Perspective*, Davis & Co. Philadelphia (1976); *Consensus Development Statement on Caesarean Section Childbirth*, NICHD, NIH, Maryland (1983).
23. Newton N. *Birth and Family J.* **1** 23-25 (1974).
24. The Patient's Association. *Can I Insist?* Leaflet, 1984. The National Association for the Welfare of Children in Hospital, 29–31 Euston Rd., London NW1 2SD, UK, and Children in Hospitals, 31 Wiltshire Park, Needham, Mass. 02192, USA will help.
25. Mason, *Arch. Gen. Psychiat.* **13** 1-8 (1965).
26. Sime, A. M. *J. Pers. Soc. Psychol.* **34** 716-724 (1976); George J. M. *et al J. Behav. Med.* **3** (1980).
27. Volicer, B. *J. Human Stress*, 28-36 (June 1978).
28. Fortin, F. and Kirouac, S. *Int. J. Nursing Studies*, **13** 11-24 (1976).
29. Volicer, B. J. *et al, J. Human Stress*, 3-13 (June 1977).
30. Johnson, J. E. In: Exploring Progress in Medical-Surgical Nursing Practice, American Nurses Assoc. N. Y. (1966).
31. Boore, J. *Prescription for Recovery*, Royal College of Nursing, London (1978).
32. Taylor, C. B. *J. Clin. Psychiat.* **43** 423-425 (1982).
33. Benson, H. *The Relaxation Response*, New York, Morrow (1975).
34. Peters, *et al, Am. J. Pub. Health*, **67** 946-959 (1977); Patel, C. *The Lancet* (10 November 1973); Beary, J. F. and Benson, *H. Psychosomatic Medicine*; 115 (March 1974).

35. Luck, S. and Kellerman S. *Whole Life Times*, 36, (June 1983).
36. Lauger, E. J. *et al, J. Exp. Soc. Psychol.*, **11** 155-165 (1975).
37. Meares, A. *Relief Without Drugs*, London, Fontana (1983); Pearce, I. *The Gate of Healing*, Neville Spearman, St. Helier, Jersey (1980).
38. Arpita, *Himalayan Institute Research Bulletin*, **4** 22 (1982).
39. Monro, R. *Yoga Biomedical Bulletin*, **1** 29 (September 1985).
40. Bishop, B. *A Time to Heal*, Severn House, UK (1985).
41. Weinsier, R. L. *Am. J. Clinical Nutrition*, (February 1979).
42. Bender, A. *British Medical J.* **288** 92-93 (1984).
43. Todd, E. *et al, Human Nutrition: Applied Nutrition*, **38A** 294-297 (1986).
44. *Prevention*, 140-145 (May 1985).
45. *Am. J. Clinical Nutrition*, (January 1985).
46. *J. Am. Dietic Association*, (December 1976); *ibid* (June 1983).
47. Basu T. K. Schorah, C. J. *Vitamin C in Health and Disease*, Croom Helm, London (1981).
48. Editorial BMJ, **212** (9 February 1974).
49. Irvin, T. T. *Surg. Gynaecol. Obst.*, **147** 49 (1978).
50. Kirschman, J. D. *The Nutrition Almanac*, McGraw Hill (1975).
51. Egger J. *et al, Lancet*, **2** 865-869 (1983); ibid, *Lancet*, **1**, 540-545 (1985).
52. Blackwood, J. and Fulder, S. *Garlic, Nature's Original Remedy*, Javelin Books, Poole, Dorset (1986).
53. Usla, B. *Research in Experimental Medicine*, **182** 7-12 (1983).
54. Rasic, J. L. and Kurmann, J. A. *Bifidobacteria and their Role*, Germany, Birkhauser Verlag (1983).
55. Bryant, M. *J. Alt. Med.* (February 1986).
56. Loiseau, *et al*, quoted in Boore, J. *Prescription for Recovery*, Royal College of Nursing, London (1978).
57. McNeil, I. *Nutrition and Health*, **2** 111-114 (1983).
58. Noak-Loebel, *et al, Prog. Food Nutrition Science*, **7** 127-131 (1983).
59. Couge, G. *et al, Reproduction, Nutrition, Development*, **20** (4A) 929-938 (1980).
60. Shorter, R. G. and Kirsner, J. B. (eds) *Gastrointestinal Immunity for the Clinician*, Grune and Stratton, N.Y. (1985).
61. Higginson, S. *Pig Farming*, April (1985).
62. Hofer, J. *Total Massage*, Grosset & Dunlop, N.Y. (1976). Downing, G., *The Massage Book*, Random House, N.Y. (1974). Kunz and Kunz, *The Complete Guide to Foot Reflexology*, Thorsons, UK (1984).
63. Lonsdale, D. *et al, Am. J. Clinical Nutrition*, **33** 205-211 (1980); Cheraskin, E. and Ringsdorf, W.M. *Psychodietetics*, Stein and Day (1975).
64. Shaw, D. M. *Br. J. Psychiatr.* **139** 580 (1981).
65. Wurtman, R. J. *Lancet*, **1** 1145-8 (1983).
66. *Am. J. Clinical Nutrition*, **39** 691 (1984).
67. Davis, A. *Let's Get Well*, New American Library, N.Y. (1980); Nutrition Search Inc. *Nutrition Almanac*, N.Y. McGraw Hill (1975).
68. *British Medical Journal*, **289** (24 November 1984).
69. Fitten, L. *et al, J. Am. Geriatr. Soc.*, **33** 294-7 (1985).

70. Dew, M. *Br. J. Clinical Practice*, **38** 394-8 (1985).
71. Fulder, S. *The Tao of Medicine*, Destiny Books, N.Y. (1982); ibid *About Ginseng*, Thorsons, Wellingborough (1980).
72. Brekhman, I. I. and Dardymov, I. V. *Lloydia*, **32** 46-51 (1969).
73. Chang, Y. S. et al, In: *Proceedings of 2nd Int. Ginseng Symposium*, Seoul, Korea (1978).
74. Brekhman, I. I. and Dardymov, I. V. *Ann. Rev. Pharmacology*, **9** 419 (1969).

CHAPTER 5

Anaesthesia Can Be Easier

Mary Young went into hospital just after her 42nd birthday for a hysterectomy because of uterine polyps. The operation was entirely successful, but:

'I discovered that something was dreadfully wrong about a day after when I tried to raise my hand to push hair off my face, and found that it flopped back, ragdoll fashion from less than shoulder height. I told the nurse who couldn't have been less interested. When I tried to lever myself to a sitting position the left arm collapsed under me. I don't mind admitting I was terrified and started trying to find out what I could do about it. Having got no sense out of the nurse I showed my gynaecologist what was happening, and he arranged that a neurologist should see me (I gathered that the surgeon operates but the patient's condition should be the concern of the anaesthetist).

'The neurologist, Dr Henry, must have known what had happened, yet he first tried to browbeat me into believing that I had an arthritic shoulder and had gone into hospital with a useless arm! When I lost my temper with him – to the best of my recollection "callow little sod" was my most charitable epithet – he admitted that possibly a nerve had been trapped during the anaesthetic and that an orthopaedic surgeon might be able to help. I nearly went wild with fear and said there was no use getting one because under no circumstances would I have another anaesthetic, and having lied to me once I did not trust his integrity, and if he was foolish enough to attempt to get in any other "so-called specialist" I should go straight through the window, second floor or not.

'Despite having routed the unspeakable Dr Henry, the rest of my stay was utterly wretched. I had lost confidence in everyone except the surgeon who came in daily to see me and put up with a lot. Imagine, too, the fun of coping with the toilet with surgical padding, panties and night clothes to deal with and only one useful hand.

'I left hospital on 1st October and saw an osteopath on the 20th. He said it was certainly a trapped nerve. After three sessions of treatment at weekly intervals I had full mobility and sensation, the thumb being the last part to return to normal feeling. I now play the piano and lute, go riding, swim twice a week, and lead a full and active life. But I wonder, is there any alternative to conventional anaesthesia?'

There *are* alternatives to anaesthesia, besides the medieval one of a bottle of brandy and some stout attendants. The newspaper pictures of stomach or heart surgery performed in China under acupuncture anaesthesia are perfectly true. The Chinese have now performed a million operations under acupuncture anaesthesia. These alternatives can also be found in the West, though limited to occasional use in dentistry, minor surgery and obstetrics. We will be discussing them later. Perhaps more important are the alternatives which can be used alongside conventional anaesthesia to help reduce unwanted effects and discomfort. Before we look at them we ought to see how anaesthesia occurs and what are its consequences.

What to Expect from Anaesthetics

Your operation is scheduled for a Thursday at 10 o'clock in the morning. What will happen?

You will probably arrive at hospital on Wednesday. On Wednesday evening the anaesthetist will drop over to see you in your ward for 5-10 minutes. He will know something of your case, but will wish to get a picture of your physical and mental fitness for the operation, particularly looking for circulatory and liver problems. He will check how anxious you are, in order to prescribe tranquillizers before the operation. Almost everyone is nervous, and research has shown that one out of two people are actually afraid of dying on the operation table. Therefore, tranquillizers are routine. A good anaesthetist may indirectly determine your mood and will postpone the operation if you are really pessimistic about your chances. If he sees that you are the kind of person who wants to know, he will give you information about the procedures.

An hour before the operation you will be given tranquillizers. These are not usually given in day-case surgery.

You will be wheeled into a waiting room and shortly before the operation you will be given drugs such as tubocurarine and atropine to relax the muscles to prevent muscle spasms, and dry up secretions.

An injection of a barbiturate such as thiopental is given to put you to sleep, and then a gaseous anaesthetic continues throughout the operation. This is usually nitrous oxide/oxygen, and halothane. The state of anaesthesia is somewhere between sleep and a coma. It is dreamless and on waking you will feel that no time has passed. Local anaesthetics such as epidurals (spinal) are preferred if possible as they are safer and cheaper. You are not normally given a choice of anaesthetic other than to be told if a local anaesthetic is possible.

The anaesthetic is timed to run out just after the operation. You are taken into a recovery room or Intensive Care Unit, and the sister will shout at you or pull your ears to wake you up. You are likely to be dizzy, faint, disorientated, nauseous and weak. But these feelings ought to pass.

The Risks of Anaesthesia

Mary suffered from one of the unexpected and unasked-for consequences of anaesthetics: a trapped nerve. It was the result of the anaesthetist failing to position her properly on the table and arrange all the piping in and around her. A dropped foot or neck dislocations can also sometimes result.

The danger of death or brain damage from anaesthesia is fortunately rather rare: about 1 in 5000 operations. It is almost always the result of anaesthetists' mistakes, such as a disconnection of a poorly connected tube.[2] It has led the *Lancet* to suggest that anaesthetists, who generally get tired and bored, should be 'grounded' after a certain number of hours, like pilots.[2] Patients at either end of their lifespan are most at risk. General anaesthetics given in the dentist's chair are more risky than in hospital, because dentists don't always ask about their patients' asthma, diabetes, liver or heart disease. These conditions can greatly increase the risks. If someone has had a heart attack within six months of an operation, he has a 1 in 20 chance of having another one just afterwards.[3]

The unborn child is, as ever, more sensitive than adults to chemicals and drugs. Assistants helping in an operating theatre have more abnormal babies simply because of the anaesthetics floating about.[4] Babies emerge from Caesarean sections significantly slower, duller and with more breathing difficulties because of anaesthetics given to the mother (see chapter 13).[5]

Yet the most common side effects of anaesthetics are psychological. The disorientation, depression, weakness and lack of healing may persist. It is not realised that mental function may take weeks to get back to normal. This shows especially in ability to solve problems, in memory, and language skills. A crossword enthusiast may find himself inextricably stumped for two months. The mental slowness is very clear to any health worker up to four days after an operation. With special tests a psychologist can distinguish those who have had a general anaesthetic for six weeks afterwards.

Local anaesthetics also have side effects, but they are much less dangerous. Of people who have epidural (spinal) anaesthetic, 3% have strong headaches afterwards. There is sometimes numbness in the limbs and problems in controlling urination. Epidurals in birth leave the mother without sensation from the waist down. Babies born to mothers who have an epidural are noticeably less reactive and responsive[6] even six weeks later.[7] They are also twice as likely to have jaundice.[8,9] This is discussed again in chapter 13.

How to Prepare Yourself for Anaesthesia

You do not have to descend helplessly into unconsciousness like someone falling down an abandoned mineshaft. There are preparations and precautions you can take beforehand.

It is worth remembering that just as the most common problems encountered with anaesthesia are mental, so the mind can resist them. Think of the classical hero cop who gets knocked out during a chase, but then gets up, shakes his head and carries on running. Anxiety, stress and exhaustion increase vulnerability to pain and the side effects of anaesthetics; while calm, confidence and energy are helpful.

Here then are some tips on easier anaesthesia.

● *Come to the operation well rested*, well fed, and well looked after. Take multivitamins for at least 10 days beforehand, especially B vitamins. Cut out alcohol and unnecessary drugs for this time to protect the liver. Try to reduce coffee and tea intake; it is known that people who consume a lot of caffeine recover more slowly from anaesthetics.

● Make use of one or other of the methods of *relaxation and confidence-building* described in Chapters 4 and 6. Request very thorough information so that you know what to expect. Your involvement in the procedure reduces the pain and helps recovery from the anaesthesia.

● *Refuse the tranquillizers* given before the operation. They make it impossible to prepare yourself and relax. You lose all clarity. They do not necessarily calm you down; instead you can feel extremely anxious and aroused, but cannot show it and cannot express it. The anxiety is frozen. This is why it is often said that tranquillizers are given to help the staff, not the patient. In addition they have side effects of their own. Many patients feel knocked out and need to recover more from tranquillizer after-effects than the anaesthetic. Tranquillizers should be taken only in extreme cases of panic when no help such as hypnosis is available.

● *Your expectations should be realistic.* Realize that you may be disorientated and depressed after the anaesthetic, and you may find writing and using language more difficult for a while. Don't try to do too much afterwards – give yourself time to recover.

● *Arrange for encouraging things to be said to you* when you are under the anaesthetic. Failing that ask for cotton wool to be put in your ears. You may not remember what went on in the operating theatre, but some part of you does register comments, especially where it concerns your fate. These can act as unconscious suggestions to affect your recovery.[10] Eve, a physiotherapist of my acquaintance, gave an anaesthetist a short poem about sleep to read to her as she went under. At first he was embarrassed to intone pastoral phrases about snoozing on a summer afternoon but now he uses the poem with everyone.

The Importance of Breathing

Proper breathing is crucial to the whole process of anaesthesia and recovery from it. As we will see in Chapter 6, instructions on breathing are sometimes given to postoperative patients to mobilize organs and passages which have become temporarily paralysed by the anaesthetic.

Yoga breathing is one of the most effective ways known of calming down the body and mind beforehand. Afterwards you can use it to expel toxic gases, clear the mind, improve recovery, increase energy and get a good night's sleep. The calming breathing exercise is alternate nostril breathing. The cleansing and recovery breathing exercises are the bellows and diaphragmatic breathing, as described in Chapter 4.

This is how yoga student Alex Barclay recently described his recovery from by-pass surgery at the Harefield Hospital:

'I awoke a few minutes later as a dulcet voice asked me to breathe deeply in and slowly out and to retain the breath when asked. I had the feeling I was back in my yoga class doing breathing exercises, but having been prewarned by the physiotherapist I knew I was in the Intensive Care Unit and now was the time to have a multitude of drain tubes removed . . . Two days later I was out of bed, in a chair practising physiotherapy, or yoga, since that was what it was . . . I have not the slightest doubt that without it I would have taken far longer to recover, and perhaps succumbed to intense postoperative depression by which I was, like everyone else, beset.[11]

Two small surveys of cancer patients who have been helped by yoga have been carried out in Cambridge, one of them at Addenbrookes hospital. Several cancer patients reported that yoga had helped them calmly prepare for surgery and recover from the anaesthetic afterwards. 'Alternative nostril breathing after injection in preparation for the theatre was so successful that I lost consciousness even before being removed from the ward . . . ' noted one patient.[12]

Hypnosis and Anaesthesia

Anaesthetists know that lower doses of anaesthetics are required with less anxious patients.[13] Relaxation leads to a faster recovery from anaesthetics and the surgery itself, less pain and narcotics, and a quicker exit from the hospital.[14] Hypnosis, or suggestion, is a very useful way of relaxing, getting back in touch with yourself and introducing a positive frame of mind, especially if you are in too much of a panic to work with self-help methods.

This can be achieved, according to medical hypnotists, by 15–20 minutes of hypnosis and relaxation in the morning before the operation.[15] The hypnotist may suggest that you will feel less pain and have a faster recovery with less side effects; that the whole operation will be a quick and easy event; and that you will soon be on your feet feeling very bright. During the hypnosis you will feel relaxed and detached. The hypnotist will suggest that you feel like that when you go into the operation and as you come out of it.

Hypnosis is not a mysterious mesmeric trance. Some medical hypnotists can induce a relaxed hypnotic state while talking about the weather. Very often you will be taken on a brief journey into childhood memories. As one elderly lady said, who was doing rather poorly after cardiac surgery, 'What was most useful, was talking about being up the valleys. I told him about where I was born.'

Hypnosis can also begin the process of mending of which the operation is but a first step. One London patient had hypnosis to prepare her for an impending colon cancer operation. During this hypnosis she discovered that she was actually very angry, mostly with her husband, and this anger was the root of her disease. Once she met the anger she could use it. She lost weight, she prepared herself for the operation, she practised self-hypnosis, and she learnt how to be a decider, not a victim. The operation was successful. She went into remission and left her husband simultaneously.

There are certain hospitals, especially in the US, where hypnosis is used as a matter of course. One such is the University of California Medical School at Sacramento. It is used more frequently with children. There are 1000 doctors trained in hypnosis in the UK, scattered about the country, although only a few hundred actually use it. Many would like to use it more but are too timid or inexperienced, so you may actually be doing them a favour if you request it. Here are some guidelines:

● Find an anaesthetist who practises hypnosis, or ask if there is anyone attached to the hospital who can do it. Alternatively ask your own hypnotist to visit you. You should tell the surgeon beforehand.

● Inform the anaesthetist that you wish to have hypnosis, and no tranquillizers.

● Try to have one or two sessions with the hypnotist before entering hospital. This can nip anxiety in the bud.

● The best time for hypnosis is an hour or two before surgery while you are in the ward.

● If you cannot find a hypnotist, find a friend or counsellor who can use images and suggestion to relax you, and who can repeat the process just before you receive the anaesthetic.

● Failing that, take a personal cassette recorder with earphones into hospital with a tape of relaxation/hypnosis which you have selected.

Anaesthesia Through Acupuncture

Until recently our knowledge of pain was little more sophisticated that of an electrician's: certain nerve fibres sent pain signals to brain pain centres. Acupuncture has changed all that.[16] The flood of reports emerging from the Far East describing acupuncture anaesthesia during surgery led to intensive research on how a prick in the thumb could reduce a pain in the head. This led to the so-called Gate Theory, which proposes that stimulation of certain nerve fibres sends blocking messages to the spine. These close the gate to pain signals on their way up the spine to the brain.[17] This theory fails to explain how acupuncture can relieve chronic pain or, indeed, how it can cure disease.

It was further discovered that there are natural painkillers, called endorphins in our brain.[18] They are there to reduce our pain feelings at critical times, for example in childbirth or in the thick of a fight. Acupuncture stimulates these brain endorphins, getting them to shut down pain over a much longer period than the usual four-hour morphine dose.[19] Acupuncture works with the body's pain relief system; narcotics replace it. This is why the more you take of them the more you need them.

The dramatic Chinese successes where patients under acupuncture anaesthesia are chatting to the surgeon during heart surgery[20] have been repeated in the West.[21] However it became clear that sedatives are often needed too, and that acupuncture can kill the pain only in some people. Besides, there are not enough well-trained experienced acupuncturists to go around. For these reasons, as well as conservatism, it is not much used in the West except in dentistry and obstetrics. In both these cases it has been shown to work with remarkable consistency.[22]

In any event there are distinct advantages in acupuncture anaesthesia. It avoids the uncomfortable side effects and potential dangers of anaesthetics, it reduces pain after the operation, there is less infection and tissue damage,[23] much less shock to the system and the patient recovers more quickly.[24] In fact acupuncture anaesthesia may be the only kind of anaesthesia possible in some patients who are suffering from shock, or are very weak, and are denied an operation with conventional anaesthesia in case it killed them. Some tips:

● Try and find an anaesthetist who is also an acupuncturist.
● It is possible to substitute acupuncture for conventional drug anaesthesia in biopsies, minor surgery such as tonsillectomy, dentistry and obstetrics.
● Under certain conditions replacing anaesthetics by acupuncture could be very important:
  If you are very weak or very ill
  If you have just had a heart attack
  If you have a weak liver
  If you have multiple allergies
  If you feel that the outcome of the operation will be poor.

● Do not worry about pain returning during the operation. The acupuncturist will constantly top up the anaesthesia by twirling the needles, and the anaesthetist will anyway be standing by.

● Your acupuncturist will test you to check if you are anaesthetisable with acupuncture. If you are not, several acupuncture treatments before the operation can make you anaesthetisable with acupuncture. It will have the added bonus of improving your health and resistance to surgery (see Chapter 6).

Another option is a newly discovered and quite remarkable substance called D-phenylalanine (D-PA). Like acupuncture it can increase the amount of endorphins in the brain.[25] Yet it is not a narcotic. It is more or less naturally occurring in the body and it can be bought without a prescription. It has the extraordinary ability to make people sensitive to acupuncture anaesthesia who would not be otherwise.[26] More about D-PA on page 86.

Pain After Surgery

'After surgery for Hodgkins Disease, when the lymph nodes were removed from my neck, I had a long treatment with radiotherapy. There was constant pain around my teeth and ear, which was referred pain from the trachea where there were no longer any nerves. Acupuncture was the only treatment which gave any relief from the pain. Painkillers didn't help but after each acupuncture treatment there were three days of relief.'

This was Susan, a 34-year-old research chemist.

Surgery is one of the most common causes of constant pain. Postoperative patients, along with migraine, slipped disc, arthritis and cancer patients, are the main clients of pain clinics. Usually the pain is unrelieved by painkillers, and narcotics are addictive. Acupuncture has been keenly accepted for chronic pain[27] because there is little else available. In fact medical acupuncture has become identified with chronic pain relief, at the expense of its therapeutic aspects.

Most pain clinics around the world now use acupuncture or one of its electrical daughters such as electroacupuncture or transcutaneous nerve stimulation (TENS). Electroacupuncture uses an electrical pulse instead of the traditional needle-twirling. It keeps to the acupuncture points, adding to them a few other electrically sensitive areas, to arrive at a treatment map on the surface of the body. Lasers are sometimes used to stimulate acupuncture points. TENS does not use acupuncture points at all, but stimulates those nerves which block pain messages. It has the advantage that you can take it home with you and keep it running while you sit by the fire.

TENS has not been fully evaluated as yet, although preliminary studies indicate that many patients using TENS find the treatment effective in pain relief.[28] It has been found to be more effective in alleviating short periods of pain than in long-term chronic pain, presumably because it acts mainly by shutting the nerve fibres' 'gate' to pain. TENS may be useful in the immediate postoperative period, reducing pain and helping to start the intestines moving again.[29] In one study at the University of Helsinki 40 patients were given TENS after dental surgery, and 40 given a pretend TENS treatment. During the second and third hour after surgery, when usually at its maximum, pain was reduced by 50% using the TENS.[30]

While it is still early days with TENS, acupuncture itself has been thoroughly evaluated for pain relief in hundreds of studies. It is generally stronger than TENS, and as it acts through the endorphins as well as the nerve gate it is capable of providing long-term as well as short-term pain relief. People suffering from chronic pain often have very low levels of endorphins.[31] This may be because of stress, disease or constitution, but the effect is the same: the endorphins have drained away and pain shows up like islands that appear when the water goes down. Chronic pain itself contributes to the depletion of endorphins, catching the sufferer in a vicious circle. There is evidence that acupuncture can break this circle by gradually restoring endorphins.[32]

Acupuncture can be very effective immediately after surgery, to help in relieving postoperative pain and hasten recovery.[33] Research has shown that psychological disturbances such as agitation, disorientation and hallucination after anaesthesia with ketamine can be prevented by ear acupuncture.[34] As a bonus to pain relief it can help directly with the side effects of anaesthetics and narcotics. As Professor Rosen, head of the anaesthetists association in the UK said recently on the BBC, 'Acupuncture can prevent postoperative sickness in a large percentage of patients.' In particular it can get your organs and intestines, partly paralysed by the surgery and anaesthetics, to start working again. This reduces nausea, headaches, gas and debility. As one obstetric surgeon reported, if electroacupuncture is given after Caesareans, 'It is astonishing how the patients can change position in the bed . . . When the patient is quiet, sitting or in bed, the pain practically does not exist and the patient feels as if there had been no surgery at all; surely a completely different condition to the one we are all familiar with when the postoperative phase is managed with the usual analgesics . . . that depress respiration and circulation, paralyse the bladder and cause nausea and vomiting, favouring development of iatrogenic complications caused and ordered by the physician himself.'[35]

With chronic postoperative pain, at least one in two people will find acupuncture helpful, and often the treatment has effects which last for months.[36] Sometimes this pain is the result of scars deep inside or on the surface, and acupuncture can help by bridging them. As two acupuncturists described to me:

'Open heart surgery involves cutting the chest. The meridians are cut. I had a patient who had a persistent cough and severe back pain after surgery. I used the TENS to bridge both sides of the cut and along with electroacupuncture treatment at the pericardian point or general confluence points the pain was greatly reduced. The advantage is that pain relief is obtained without addiction to ever stronger painkillers with their side effects.'

'I get a lot of cases of pain after operations and this is mostly the result of scarring, especially where there has been more than one operation in the same place, such as the back. In such cases I use acupuncture points around the scars and the first point on the meridian above the scar. It is like shunting electricity around a blockage.'

Other Ways to Reduce Chronic Postoperative Pain

Hypnosis is another drugless option for pain relief. It is often available in pain clinics, including one or two NHS pain clinics in the UK. Hypnosis can help you live with your pain by fundamentally changing your attitude to it. It, too, is capable of increasing the level of endorphins, as are placebos. The hypnotist can implant suggestions for positive enjoyment of life, for comfort and for well-being. Hypnosis is as effective as acupuncture for short-term pain.[37] However like acupuncture there are some people for whom it does not work well. The more suggestible you are, the more hypnosis can help you.

For chronic pain conditions hypnosis needs to be reinforced regularly. The best way to do this is by self-hypnosis, which is usually taught by the professional hypnotherapist while the patient is under hypnosis. This kind of approach has proven value in pain from serious or terminal diseases such as cancer, where acupuncture does not always work, and where a psychological approach is more important to the patient's overall comfort.[38] It has not been tested in postoperative pain and does not have the power of acupuncture to help in pain from repeated surgery and from internal scars.

Meditation is similar. It should be taught properly and many chronic pain patients have been helped by TM (transcendental meditation), autogenics and other methods. The relief may be long lasting. In one study relief from chronic pain was reported 15 months after a 10-day intensive meditation instruction.[39] Meditation and self-hypnosis can be recommended to increase wellbeing and raise the pain threshold.

Finally we return to D-PA, a remedy which is receiving eulogies from pain patients:

> 'If I believed in magic I would say this phenylalanine stuff *is* magic. Whatever it is, it works. It got me off drugs and got rid of, oh, I'd say, about 80-90% of the pain. What used to be terrible pain is now only a minor annoyance, I hardly notice it. I lost all the weight I gained because of the drugs, I'm not nauseous any more, and I can see straight.'[40]

D-PA works by blocking the removal of endorphins, which like all body components are continually being made and destroyed. The result is high levels of endorphins, which give pain relief over a long period.[25] While normal painkillers have an effect lasting for a few hours, a single dose of D-PA lasts for several days. The pain-relieving effect is slow to begin – it takes up to a month to build up. But then it stays.[41] It is extremely safe, being a mirror image or right-hand version of L-phenylalanine, an amino acid which is part of our daily diet. D-PA can be taken as part of a pain-relief programme. It is still somewhat experimental. Doctors with an interest in pain are likely to have heard of it by the time this book comes out. There are already some hospitals in Scandinavia where D-PA is prescribed along with painkillers after surgery in order to obtain 'a totally painless postoperative period.'[42]

REFERENCES

1. 400,000 operations had been performed up to 1971 (*People's China*, October 1971). Various authorities suggest 1m as the total to date.
2. Editorial, *Lancet*, **1** 593 (1979).
3. Editorial, *Lancet*, **2** 1350 (1978).
4. Weitz, M. *Health Shock*, p. 32 David & Charles, Newton Abbot (1980).
5. DHSS Report into Confidential Enquiries into Maternal Deaths in England and Wales, 1970–1972 (Report on Health and Social Subjects No. 11, 1975); see also references Chapter 13.
6. Scanlon, J. W. *et al, Anaesthesiology*, **40** 121-8 (1974); Rosefsky, *New Eng. J. Med*, **278** 530-3 (1968).
7. Rosenblatt, *et al, Brit. J. Obst. Gynaecol.*, **88** 407-413 (1981).
8. Wood, B. *et al, Arch. Dis. Child*, **54** 111-115 (1979).
9. Richards, M. *New Scientist*, 847-849 (21 September 1978); O'Driscoll, K. *Brit. J. Anaesthesia*, **47** 1053 (1975), see also Chapter 13.
10. Goldman, L. *Awareness Under Anaesthesia*, Ph.D Thesis, Churchill College Cambridge UK (1986).
11. Alex Barclay *Yoga Today*, Summer 1986.

12. Monro, R. *Yoga Biomedical Bulletin*, **1** 35, June 1985.
13. Williams, J. L. *et al, Psychophysiology*, **12** 50-54 (1973).
14. Hayward, D. J. *Information: A Prescription Against Pain*, Whitefriars Press, London (1975).
15. Scotts, D. L. *Hospital Hypnosis for Anaesthestists*, publisher unknown.
16. Lewith, G. T. and Kenyon, J. N. *Soc. Sci. Med.*, **19** 1367-1378 (1984).
17. Wall, P. and Sweet, W. H. *Science*, **155** 108-9 (1967); Nathan, P. W. *Brain*, **99** 123-158 (1976); Melzack R. *The Puzzle of Pain*, Penguin, London (1973).
18. Bishop, B. *Phys. Ther.*, **60** 13-38 (1980); Way (ed.) *Endogenous and Exogenous Opiate Agonists and Antagonists*, Pergamon Press, Oxford (1979).
19. Cheng, R. S. & Pomeranz, B. *Life Sciences*, **26** 613-639 (1979); Clement-Jones, V. *et al, Lancet*, **2** 946-948 (1980).
20. Third People's Hospital, Shanghai Medical College and Hunan Medical College, *Chin. Med. J.*, **8** 453-466 (1974).
21. Herget, H. G. *et al, Der Anaesthetist*, **25** 223 (76).
22. Tany, M. *et al, Am. J. Acupuncture*, **2** 287-294 (1975); Craciun, T. and Csiki, A, *Am. J. Acupuncture*, **6** 127 (1978).
23. Matsumoto, T., *Experimental Acupuncture Anaesthesia – Acupuncture for Physicians*, N. Y. Charles C. Thomas (1974). Roscia, L. *Am. J. Chinese Med.*, **1** 325 (1973).
24. Dept. Anaesthesiology, Anwhei Medical College, *Chin. Med. J.*, **2** 95-100 (1973).
25. Ehrenpreis, S. *et al, Adv. in Pain Res. and Ther.*, **3** 479-487 (1979); Cheng, R. S. S. and Pomeranz, B. *Brain Res.* **177** 583-587 (1979).
26. Hyodo, M. *Pain*, S181 (S1) (1981); Takeshige, C. *et al*, In: Takagi, H. and Simon, E. J. (eds.) *Avances in Endogenous and Exogenous Opioids*, Tokyo, Kodansha-Elsevier (1982).
27. Editorial *Brit. Med. J.,* **283**, 746-8 (1981); Wei, L. Y. *Am. J. Chinese Med.*, **7** 53-75 (1979); Peking Children's Hospital, *Chinese Med. J.*, **1** 369-374 (1975); Coan *et al, Am. J. Chinese Med.*, **8** 181-9 (1980).
28. Taylor, *et al, Pain*, **11** 233 (1981).
29. Solomon, *et al, Surgery*, **87** 142 (1980); Pike, P. K. H., *Anaesthesia*, **33** 165-71 (78); Hymes, A. C. *et al, Surgical Forum*, **24** 447-9 (1973).
30. Ihalainen, U. & Perkki, K. *Acup & Electrotherap. Res.*, **5** 313-321 (1980).
31. Akil, H. *Science*, **201** 463-5, (1978).
32. Nappi, G. *et al, Acup. Electrotherap.*, **7** 93-104 (1982); Gang, L. *et al, In National Symposium of Acupuncture, Moxibustion, and Acupuncture Anaesthesia*, 447, Peking, (1979).
33. Sung, Y. G. *et al, Anaesth. Analg. Curr. Res.*, **56** 473-8 (1977).
34. Ceccherelli, F. *et al, Acup. Electrotherap. Res.*, **6** 255-264 (1981).
34. Rodriguez, R. *Am. J. Acupuncture*, **6** 123-6 (1978).
36. Richardson, P. H. and Vincent C. A. *Pain*, **24** 15-40 (1986).
37. Stern, J. A. *et al, Ann. N. Y. Acad. Sci.*, **296**, 175-193 (1977).
38. Ament, P. *J. Medicine*, 233-240 (1982); Meares, A. *Relief Without Drugs*, London Fontana (1970).
39. Kabat-Zinn, J. *et al, Behav. Med.*, **8** 163 (1985).
40. Fox, A. and Fox, B. *Let's Live*, 10 (January 1985).

41. Budd, K. *Pain*, S95 (S1) 1981; Balagot R. C. and Ehrenpreis S. *Anaesthesiology*, **51** S231 (1979).
42. Pontinen, P. J. *Acup. and Electrotherap. Res.*, **8** 73 (1983).

CHAPTER 6

Surgery

At Knifepoint

'I'm sure it's nothing, but just to be on the safe side we'll have it out.'
Something about these comforting, enticing words makes the hair stand on
the back of the neck.

Surgery is the best of modern medicine: the highly skilled professionals,
the elaborate technical backup, the detailed, concentrated knowledge of
the offending anatomy, the wizardry of repairing damaged tissues, the
superb management of large numbers of people, and the computerized
monitoring equipment. If the hospital is the temple of medicine, the
operating theatre is its altar.

Yet by the same token it is the worst of medicine: the highly skilled professionals have no real contact with the patient and little understanding of
the root causes of the illness, the technical backup causes stress to the
patient and dehumanization so that full recovery is delayed or prevented.
The concentration on an anatomical piece means that the patient himself is
a mere carrier of his problem – 'the prostate in bed 7'. The management is
at the expense of communication, the computers at the expense of
touching, the repair mentality elbows out prevention and instruction.

Surgery is often a vital life-saving procedure. There would be little
argument about the 20% of surgery that is emergency work. An emergency
is an emergency. But the other 80% of surgery, however brilliant, is often
unnecessary, beset by unexpected complications, and accompanied by an
apparent ignorance of the feelings of the patient and the basic requirements
for a return to long-term health and wellbeing.

In this chapter I will discuss the evidence for this statement, and help you
to recognize and avoid unnecessary surgery, to choose the right procedure
and the right person to do it, and to reduce the risks and hasten your
recovery.

Destructive Zeal: Unnecessary Surgery and Its Sequel

Strange as it may seem, surgical procedures are rarely scientifically
assessed before introduction. Only occasionally, long after they are in

widespread use, are evaluations ever made. The results have often been quite negative and it has been shown that many of the patients would have recovered without such assaults.[1]

In the US surgeons are paid for each operation. This has led to so much unnecessary surgery that a US Senate Committee was set up to investigate it. They reported that 2.4 million unnecessary operations were performed each year causing 12,000 deaths and wasting $4 billion.[2] Less guarded opinions, such as that of the heart surgeon Robert G. Schneider in his book *When to Say No to Surgery*, estimate more than 6 million unnecessary operations per year.[3] Where surgeons are paid a fixed salary the number of operations drops by two thirds, meaning that in two thirds of the cases the surgeon was performing the operation for his own rather than the patient's benefit. Just the existence of a hospital committee to check whether surgery is necessary or not has been found to reduce appendix removals by two thirds.[4]

In the UK paying surgeons for each operation would be as unthinkable as paying policemen for each arrest. There is therefore half the amount of surgery than in the US. Even so, 20,000 useless appendix removals are performed each year.[5]

Some operations swing in and out of fashion in an alarming way, showing that yesterday's doctors fancy them but today's patients don't need them. For example three quarters of all British children had their tonsils removed in the 1930s. Now we know that children without tonsils suffer as much if not more from infections as those with them.[6] Would the children have submitted, despite the ice creams afterwards, if they had known that they would be three times more likely to suffer from polio,[7] and have a four-fold increase in the risk of a cancer, Hodgkin's Disease?[8] It is now clear that tonsils are inflamed only because they are trying to do their job of filtering out the smoke and pollution; tonsils are removed much more frequently from children whose parents smoke.[9] Apart from a few cases where the tonsils are actually stopping the breath, removing the tonsils is a bit like smashing the sink if the drains are blocked. Yet 90,000 tonsilectomies are still performed in the UK and 250,000 in the US every year.

One current fashion is high-tech tests that are mini-operations requiring a general anaesthetic. One example is laparoscopy, inspection of the inside of the abdomen by a tube inserted through the stomach wall. It is often ordered very casually, like opening the car bonnet to take a look inside.

Which Are the Unnecessary Operations?

Some operations may be necessary at certain times with certain people. The instructions later on in this chapter on how to restrain the surgeon and reduce the risks will help you to decide if an operation is really necessary.

The Most Common Unnecessary Operations

Operation	Reasons for Doubt
Appendix removal	Three quarters of all appendices removed in Germany found normal.[10]
Back operations	Surgery often has no advantage over safer treatments e.g. physiotherapy. *Lancet* says 60% of operations unnecessary.[11]
Biopsy	If for cancer, may spread it.[12] Can sometimes be done by your GP.
Breast removal	Removal of whole breast does not increase survival over removal of lump only[13,14], or quarter of breast.[15] Review of 8,000 cases show no differences in survival between any of the procedures.[16] Stress of surgery can spread the cancer.[17] Surgeons now confused[18] and patients turning to alternatives.[19] Breast removal traumatic: quarter of all patients suicidally depressed.
Heart By-pass	Recovery slow. Scarring and depression common. Patients do not live longer after operation unless blockage severe.[20] European Coronary Surgery Study Group showed benefits marginal if at all.[21]
Circumcision	*British Medical Journal* says its safer at home than in hospital.[22]
Gallstone removal	One in 30 elderly die from operation.[23] Leaves scars and pain. But 'quiet' stones often removed unnecessarily.[24] New safe ultrasonic method available.
Heart and Kidney Transplants	Russian roulette. Alternative methods can also save hearts and kidneys.
Hernia	Four times more dangerous to have operation than to go without.[25]
Hysterectomy	Only one in five clinically fully justified in US where ½ million performed p.a.[26] 30% of cases infected[27], 40% depressed.[28,29]
Tonsils and Adenoids removal	Not necessary except where danger of blockage.[30]
Tympanostomy (Ear Drum Puncture and Drainage)	An unnecessary fashion, like tonsil removal. Blockages treatable by diet.
Shaving before surgery	Creates more infection than leaving hair, according to *Lancet*.[31]

On the previous page is a table of the most common unnecessary procedures. If your impending operation is one of these it should make you doubly alert to the possibility that you have been recruited into undergoing a procedure which is not worth the risks.

The Side Effects of Surgery

Mary Matthews, a poor strained single mother has been in and out of hospital with Systemic Lupus Erythematosis (SLE) and psoriasis. She has been on steroids continually and uncomplainingly for 14 years. One day she came in with pain and a distended stomach. She had three laparoscopies which were inconclusive. Then a gynaecologist took over her case and opened up her abdomen to examine the uterus. Finding nothing he sewed her up and passed her case on to a liver specialist, who finally diagnozed that the abdominal swelling was a symptom of SLE, something which could have been looked up in any medical paperback. The steroids may also have contributed to it.

Now, as she was on steroids, her operation wound did not heal. She was in pain, and developed a hernia. This caused an intestinal blockage which was repaired in emergency surgery by a first-class surgeon. But she was so weakened by the disease and the operations that, though she went on holiday after the operation, she was soon back in hospital with further abdominal problems where, after a while, she caught pneumonia and died.

There are more complications and risks of surgery than are realized. Those who partially recover may remain vulnerable, semi-sick, depressed and suffering from 'unrelated' health problems which go unrecorded. The average risk of dying from non-emergency surgery is 1 in 100, but the fact that 30% of women who have hysterectomies never have sex again remains a risk that surgeons are unlikely to talk about.[26]

The risks are greater the longer the operation. They depend on the type of operation, the place where it occurs and the surgeon in charge. For example at one London hospital 1 in 20 patients had infected wounds after orthopaedic surgery, six times the rate of a smaller hospital in the north of the country.[32]

The risks derive from:

Anaesthesia. One death in 5,000, but more risk for the old, the very young, and those with heart problems (see chapter 5).

Infections. Many people pick up an infection during surgery – for example more than 30% of women who have hysterectomies.[27,31] In the UK 3,000 people die from such infections per year, and long illnesses are much more common.

Blood transfusions. Diseases (such as AIDS or hepatitis), errors and complications cause about one death in 9,000 operations and more illness.

Haemorrhage. Internal bleeding during or after surgery is the major cause of death.

Blood clots that wander, shock, slips-of-the-knife, or wrong operations are other kinds of physical risks.

Scarring. This is the major cause of postoperative pain, discomfort and ill-health which may last for years. It is often unrecognized by the medical profession.

Psychological complications. These can be a sad sequel to surgery and just as crippling as physical complications, yet they are rarely taken very seriously. Minor brain damage can be quite common in cardiac surgery, arising from toxic residues of anaesthetics, sterilizing gases or plastic tubes, and clots or bubbles in the circulation. Hysterectomies are notorious for causing long bouts of depression, and even Caesareans can leave a mother inexplicably depressed for months.

Unknown causes. Fifteen women recently had minor surgery without obvious problems. After they awoke from the anaesthetic they became confused, demented, and lapsed into a coma. Six died and the rest are disabled. Doctors are not sure of the reason but, according to the *New York Times* of 11th June 1986, it may be that shock and fear, coupled with the drugs and the intravenous drip, upset the self-regulating mehanisms of the body. Milder cases also occur.

Restraining the Surgeon and Selecting the Treatment

When you are first recommended by your doctor for an operation two doors are open to you. The first is oiled with encouragement; it leads to a well-used passageway that slopes gently downhill. You are transferred from friendly doctor to smooth surgeon, are booked efficiently into hospital and shunted into bed. You sign the forms, are wheeled to the theatre, lose a bit of your anatomy, and are drip-fed afterwards. But on this path you are both a guest and a victim. It requires you to lose yourself, your voice, your control, your choices.

The longer you walk on this path the more risk there is that you will lose your health. The path may turn gradually into a Via Dolorosa.

The other door is more difficult to enter. You face an uphill climb requiring work, independence and watchfulness, and which may involve misunderstandings and even hostility. You have to keep hold of your freedom, your choices, your sense of protection. Yet this path is more likely to be that of survival and recovery. Apart from emergency operations, when you are literally rushed through the first door, the choice is yours.

To go through the survival door you need all the help you can get. You may be worried, confused, tired, ill and frightened, and you have the job of negotiating your way through a maze peopled by smooth, overconfident and determined professionals. But you have several big advantages:

- *Your sense of survival* which made you want to go the harder road in the first place.
- *Your rights and freedoms* as a citizen and consumer.
- *Your inner strength* and natural resilience.
- *Their obligation* to provide you with a service at minimum risk.
- *Your allies*—friends, family, self-help groups and even nurses.

You must learn how to marshall these advantages and make your journey through the survival door as easy as possible.

Stage 1. Learning and Preparation

Gather Resources

The surgeon holds up the X-rays, and says: 'Yes, I'm afraid it is . . .' (that word you hoped he wouldn't say). 'I'll book you in next week to the hospital. You'd better make arrangements with your work for a month off.' You are a mass of confusion, depression and possibly pain. The first thing to do is to cool down and take a break. In any event you should not enter an operation under panic and stress. It is as important to take time off work now as for the operation itself. You have things to do and you must relax, calm down and do them. Non-emergency surgery is rarely so urgent that you cannot take time to prepare yourself. If necessary, ask the surgeon what precise risks you will run by delaying the operation. You may need anything up to a month for the next steps.

Understand your medical problems. Read about your problem in popular medica books, in the Physicians Desk Reference and in health magazines. Go to your library or a medical library. Discuss it with medical and non-medical friends.

You need to know:

- Whether the diagnosis you have been given really seems to fit your situation.
- What are the existing options for treatment?
- What are the chances of success with each treatment, and what are the side effects?
- Why the disease may have appeared in you at this time?
- Whether it is part of a pattern of recurring disease in your life.
- Whether there are suitable alternative non-conventional treatment methods.

Contact self-help groups. You are not alone. Find self-help groups from health education, consumer and public information services. For example there will be self-help groups of mastectomy patients (see Appendix). Ask them what are the best and safest treatments, hospitals and surgeons.

Examine complementary medicine. Can you avoid conventional surgery and medical treatment altogether by seeking complementary medical treatment? Find out if your condition is amenable to dietary, acupuncture, osteopathic/chiropractic, psychotherapeutic, homeopathic or herbal treatment. Most people can be helped by these methods. Talk to people who have used complementary medicine and discuss your case with one or more practitioners. The extra cost may save you a great deal more later.

Stage 2. Back to the Professional

Ask the Right Questions

Now ask for an appointment with your surgeon, and make sure that it is long enough before the operation date to take further steps with the calmness and information won from stage 1. You may not have all the answers, but you know some of the questions, and you are not prepared to swallow the diet of bland, off-the-shelf assurances that such interviews often consist of. You want it straight. 'Don't concern yourself with details,' or any other evasive or dismissive approach should be dealt with by a polite request to be informed of all the relevant facts, procedures and outcomes, in order that you can make an intelligent decision on the treatment. The way to do this is described in Chapter 2.

You have in the case of surgery an extra means of ensuring the dialogue you need beyond those described in that chapter.

Before surgery you must sign a form of consent, which states that you have been fully informed. Tell the surgeon: 'How can I give informed consent if you do not provide me with information?'

Studies exist which demonstrate that if patients are fully informed before surgery, they enter it with less stress, and after it they have less pain, fewer complications and a faster recovery.[34] You should state that you need the answer to your questions so as to be less anxious during and after the event.

Your trust in your doctor and surgeon is important for your recovery. But this trust must come *after* you have made your decisions. While you assess treatment options it would be wise to be wary.

As Robert Mendelsohn advises:[26]

● *Don't assume* that the operation is necessary.
● *Don't be deceived* by a well-polished air of confidence.
● *Don't assume* that all the treatment choices have been considered.
● *Don't assume* that the surgery will actually make you feel better.
● *Don't assume* that the surgeon cannot make mistakes.

You should ask the questions and approach the consultant as described in Chapter 4. In addition ask him these five questions:

1. What is the complication rate for this procedure?
2. How many of these operations have you done? (If under 10 don't use this surgeon/consultant.)
3. How long will it take me to recover, and how long to be back at work?
4. What should I do after the operation to promote recovery?
5. Will you do the surgery yourself or will you just supervise?

The competence of the surgeon is vital to the success of the operation. A survey of 1,500 complications by the American College of Surgeons in 95 US hospitals found that three quarters of the complications were due to surgeon errors. You need the best. Therefore if it is turns out that:

● He will not be doing the surgery himself (in the case of private medicine);

● or he does not give satisfactory answers to the other questions;

● or he cannot be persuaded to give you the information that you need;

● or he 'feels' all wrong and you would be very nervous under his hands;

then you can change him. But don't change your specialist for frivolous reasons, i.e. that the young Dr Jones seems more friendly than the horrid old fellow you seem to have ended up with. You can go about changing him as described in Chapter 4.

Second opinions are necessary in the case of serious surgery, or if you are not happy about the answers you receive. Insurance companies will usually pay for them, and sometimes you can get them on the NHS if you ask the consultant.

Choose a second opinion surgeon in the way described in Chapter 4, either directly or on the advice of another practitioner by private arrangement. In the US there is a Second Surgical Opinion Hotline at (800) 638 6388.

The Anaesthesiologist/Anaesthetist

Try to see the anaesthetist well beforehand, instead of his usual 5-minute visit the night before the operation, when you are just trying to get your bearings in hospital. Ask him which anaesthetic and why? Can it be done with a local? What are the risks? Will he do it personally or will he leave it mostly to a specially trained nurse?

Entering the Arena

You have decided to have the operation; there is no other choice, and the benefits are worth the risks. So far, so good. Now you have to concentrate on getting the best out of your treatment, physically, emotionally and psychologically.

Your Rights and Surgery

Firstly you should know where you stand (or more accurately lie) in case things do go drastically wrong. Despite any pressure put on you, no one can force you to sign anything, to do anything or to receive any treatment. If you are not getting the procedure agreed on previously, you can refuse it. However the hospital can also refuse to treat you—you do not have a right to a particular treatment, you only have a right to competent treatment. Under the NHS you have no right to a particular surgeon, but you do of course if you have paid for him. You do not lose your rights by signing consent forms or other forms.

Your Consent

A consent form must be presented to you before the operation. This is in addition to any general consent to treatment you may have signed on admission to the hospital. The consent form is often, through carelessness, given just before the operation when you are too nervous or drugged to know how to handle it. Therefore ask your houseman or intern for it beforehand.

● The consent form must describe exactly the procedure you agreed upon beforehand with your surgeon.
● It will have a blanket clause of this type:
● 'I also consent to such further or alternative operative measures as may be found to be necessary during the course of the operation, and to the administration of a general, or other anaesthetic for any of these purposes.'

As a wise consumer, wary of unnecessary surgery, you may want to strike this out. You are free to do so.

● You may choose to strike out the clause (in teaching hospitals) permitting observers and spectators.
● You may strike out the clause permitting disposal of material removed during the operation, for example it you want a second opinion on a biopsy sample.
● Do not sign that you have been fully informed unless that is the case.

How to Deal With Stress and Anxiety Before Operations

Hospital is a place where, strangely, you are stressed to be healed, and surgery is the most stressful of all hospital experiences.[35] Unlike a soldier who is wounded in battle but in the heat of the moment hardly realises it, surgery leaves you open to the knife, aware of the consequences, in unfamiliar surroundings, without control over yourself, with your very life and integrity in the hands of strangers whose competence you can only guess at. You are very frightened of the possibility of pain, damage or even death, and there is usually no one to hold your hand through the experience.

There has been a great deal of research showing that the more anxious a patient is, the more difficult is the operation; there is extra pain, and longer recovery and recuperation. For example a study on patients who had dental surgery found that if they were very anxious, there was more tissue damage, which healed slowly. They also complained of more pain and had to be given added anaesthetic. Anxiety breeds discomfort; as the authors concluded, 'expectations about postoperative suffering did seem to act like a self-fulfilling prophecy'.[37] The anticipation of surgery releases a flood of stress hormones which reduce resistance, and the longer patients wait in hospital for an operation the weaker they become. Tranquillizers are given just before an operation. However the stress may be there for hours or days previously, and the tranquillizers have the unfortunate result of adding confusion to the stress, preventing you, inside the fog, from coping with it. The existence of tranquillizers has also permitted doctors to escape from the problem of psychological preparation for surgery. Hospital doctors' knowledge about stress or anxiety and its consequences is minimal. Nurses know a little more. You will have to help yourself.

Confidence

You have prepared yourself, you have chosen the treatment, and you have done your best. Now leave your doubts behind, they are no longer useful. Instead you need the confidence that you will be well. It is up to the doctor to play his part, and your body to do likewise. You can relax and give them both the trust they need to do their job. It is not fruitful to battle with doctors at the best of times, and the operating theatre is undoubtedly the last place to do so. Instead, encourage the doctors and share with them the burden of getting you well.

This confidence may seem like a will o'the wisp if you are sick, depressed and worried. However there are tricks to elicit it. One academic I knew was agonizing for ages whether or not to have a heart bypass operation. Careful preparation of the kind we have discussed gave him the answer that he should have it, as he didn't want to go through life 'waiting for the other shoe to drop'. His wife, who is a psychologist, told him to write everything down, both before the operation and afterwards; what he felt, what he saw, what were his values, his reactions. This made him involved and important, and built his confidence.

Information

Jennifer Boore, Professor of Nursing at the University of Coleraine in Northern Ireland has written a short book on a study she carried out. It is clinical research with a heart, if that is not a contradiction in terms. Forty patients about to undergo gall bladder and hernia operations were sympathetically prepared with information about the pre-operative medication, the transfer to the theatre, the drips, anaesthetics, tubes and procedures, and the likely feelings and pain afterwards. Forty other patients having these operations had a general chat instead. The group who were fully forewarned were much less anxious and had less stress hormones in their blood. Only six out of 40 had an infection in their wounds or urinary system afterwards compared with 15 of the uninformed. At the fifth day after the operation those who had information began to shoot ahead physically and mentally.[38] It is the responsibility of the nursing practitioner' concluded Professor Boore, 'to ensure that such instruction is included in pre-operative care of the surgical patient.' Tell it to your nurse!

Information gives you realistic expectations which reduce your worry of the unknown. In a classic book on medical stress Professor Janis calls this 'psychological innoculation', a taste of the experience so that you can get ready for it.[39] Such attention to patients undergoing hernia operations or heart catheterization reduced the need for drugs and drip-feeding after the operation and hastened recovery.[34,36] Surgeons ought to tell you that it can take you many months to be fully back on your feet after a Caesarean or hysterectomy so at least depression is not added to debility. However surgeons are usually too busy for these details, so get them from the houseman or intern who will be keeping in touch with you, and from the nurses.[41]

Unfortunately you are dependent on others for information, so you may not get it. You may also be the type who definitely doesn't want to know the details but prefers to pass through the experience in blissful ignorance. However, there is much more you can do about stress.

Relaxation

June Pressman, a 30-year-old somewhat nervous woman living in Manchester, entered hospital for an operation for an enlarged infected appendix. On the operating table surgeons found the abscess to be on the stomach wall itself rather than the appendix. They inserted a drain, but for three months the infection did not clear up, and caused her much discomfort. She says:

'I came to hospital on Thursday afternoon and tried to sleep early, as I was exhausted from worrying about my own health and about my mother who was completely dependent on me. Though ill, and in pain, I could hear the birds outside which then made me cry as I felt cut off. I couldn't relax. They gave me a sleeping pill and eventually I dropped off but the next morning I was thick and woozy. The junior surgeon came to give me a few words and write up my notes, which was good, but the anaesthetist didn't visit me as he had promised even for the pre-med. The consultant came by and asked me how was the operation, which I hadn't yet had, and these confusions made me terribly tense and panicky. They wheeled me through a waiting area to the theatre, and the surgeon waved, but the theatre staff were very impersonal and clanked about like dustmen. The pre-med made me feel like a zombie and even more confused and as things weren't going according to plan

I became terribly upset. I remember chewing my lips when they gave me the injection. I awoke in the recovery room crying and sobbing and after a few words with a gowned someone or other, I was wheeled back to my ward. I was drained, shattered, depressed and I wanted to die.'

Perhaps because of the stress, her recovery was painful and prolonged. During this period a strong determination crystallized inside her never to go through such an experience again. The infection didn't clear up and she was told she would have to have another operation. She went to a psychotherapist:

'He told me that the illness is itself just a symptom, and that we need to get to the bottom of it. He used hypnotherapy and deep relaxtion to go back to my childhood and through this I realized that I was torn by guilt for being such a naughty and ungrateful child. It came out in a great deal of anxiety and nervous caring for my mother, now disabled, which made me ill. We made a tape together which teaches me to enter a deeply relaxing space where I can feel and be comfortable with all parts of myself. I am now confident enough to go back again for more surgery to remove damaged intestinal tissue.'

This time, armed with her tape and a personal cassette recorder, she is in charge. She has work to do. She is relaxed, ready for the treatment, understanding what it is, what is required of her and what the doctors have to do. She does not need to fight them either, for she knows she will be well, and she is.

In a careful study at the University of Kentucky at Lexington Dr John F. Wilson found that if patients were given a relaxation training tape before their hysterectomies or gall bladder operations, they played it keenly before surgery and at least once a day afterwards. They were able to leave the hospital a day earlier than a matched group of patients who were given a general background tape about the hospital. They also had less pain. Four out of five said that the tape was helpful and they would use it again if they were hospitalized.[42]

Relaxation, as we have seen in Chapter 4, involves moving progressively through the body tensing and relaxing each part, telling your body, your organs and your tissues to let go.[43] This lifts tension and anxiety, reduces pain, enables more blood to reach the injury, and, most important, relaxes the tense muscles around the surgical wound to help healing. Remember to learn it before you go to hospital, and take a tape with you to help you to concentrate when you are disturbed or in pain.

A Friend Indeed
I asked a number of patients, alternative practitioners and nurses what would be the greatest single help before and just after an

operation. Most said: a good friend. People think of visitors coming after it is all over. A true friend is needed even more before it begins. But there may be a difference between visitors and a true friend. Visitors can be like a bunch of seagulls wheeling and squawking around a piece of fish. A true friend is a source of encouragement, sympathy, and tireless assistance. 'When she couldn't walk to the toilet, I was her spine, when she despaired, I was her hope, when she needed peace, I was her guardian,' was how someone described her care for her mother in hospital.

Hospitals don't always get along with visitors, but they ought to, because of the way they can reduce anxiety and stress. Researchers in the US have demonstrated how visitors can promote recovery. 'Visitors may have reassured the patient about her impending surgery. Visitors could also have been a distraction . . . a type of relaxation,'[45] was how one study saw it. The reaction to a friendly face can be dramatic. This is how Penny Brohn described her rescue during a lumpectomy under local anaesthetic[19]:

> 'My lump didn't want to part company with me and stubbornly refused to co-operate with the surgeon's efforts. I bled a lot, everybody swabbed. The frown lines around the eyes over the mask deepened, the pain grew worse and worse. More and more anaesthetic made no difference, not to the breast that is, although I was almost paralysed down the left-hand side for hours afterwards. Nasty clinking, clanking noises. More pain, more difficult to cope with. Relax, breathe properly, relax. Dear God, help me, I can't bear it. Then comfort; the theatre sister, sitting next to me, putting her arms around me, murmuring encouragement, barking and snapping at my tormentors. I love her.'

Hypnosis and Healing Before and After Surgery

Hypnosis
Very often a person who has surgery is in a crisis – emotional, energetic, social crisis. The crisis takes away the will to help oneself. It could lead to a difficult operation and a slow recovery. One hypnotist I know visited his friend who had been in an accident and was carried unconscious into the theatre. He awoke from the anaesthetic shouting and fearful, tearing the stitches. The hypnotist hypnotized his friend (who did not recognize him) by talking about rest, warmth and comfort. The friend slept immediately. Later he implanted suggestions of a speedy recovery, and this occurred.

Hypnosis can cut through the panic and open the gate to inner resources. Doctors in the UK use it mostly for pain relief, relaxation, for psychosomatic disease such as migraine and in reducing anxiety.[46,33] It is very valuable with children before surgery or dentistry, both because they are such good subjects, and because they are much more vulnerable to the fear, shock and pain produced by medical treatment.[49] Hypnosis before operations is no longer the rare peculiarity it once was.

Hypnosis merges into relaxation at one end and trance at the other. It is a method of bypassing the thinking, worrying mind and reaching down to deeper layers. Often this is quite simply done by suggesting relaxation, by pictures, numbers or repetitive sounds or images. It goes beyond deep relaxation by implanting specific suggestions in the unconscious mind. People vary in their suggestibility, and it seems that those who are suggestible will be able to achieve the more dramatic results produced by instructions given while in deep trance. But most people will be helped by hypnosis – one consultant said that hypnosis allowed 90% of minor fractures to be set in a casualty department without any anaesthetic at all.[48] In the special conditions of panic and fear before operations you are actually more quickly hypnotizable because you are more open to help. For this reason any army doctor can often hypnotize a wounded soldier with little more than the pass of a hand. The hypnotist will suggest that you relax, are confident, feel less pain, and will recover quickly afterwards. All these advantages have in fact been shown to result from pre-operative hypnosis.[46]

It would be best to undergo hypnosis once or twice before you enter hospital if you want to use it pre-operatively, as it is important to build a rapport with the hypnotist. He can also teach you to do it yourself. You should seek permission of your consultant or surgeon to bring a medical hypnotist to see you. Lay hypnotists can be brought in as a 'friend' or 'counsellor' if the surgeon or anaesthetist baulks at the idea.

Spiritual Healing

Spiritual healing is an active transmission of therapeutic energy by a trained or gifted healer, or group of healers, to a patient. It can help to re-integrate the patient's spiritual, psychological and physical aspects, give a boost to his self-healing capacity, and increase overall comfort. It is often achieved by a concentrated form of touching. After surgery healing could hasten recovery and repair. Indeed, where slow recovery creates a life-or-death situation, healing can occasionally make a dramatic impact.[50]

A less obvious function is to repair the damage of surgery on a subtle level so that it will not recur as pain or ill-health later on. This is how one healer put it:

'Surgery can be emotionally draining, especially if it is the removal of part of the body to which there is a strong emotional tie, such as hysterectomy or mastectomy. This can lead to chronic tiredness and depression. I 'see' this damage of surgery as a hole in the aura. I simply darn the hole like darning an old sock, the energy drain is plugged and the patient recovers.'

Healing can accomplish something else – it can work on a suture to prevent scarring. A very great deal of post-surgical pain, which can last for years, is due to the scars and the tissue memory of the damage. Through healing, tensions are released, circulation improves and nerves are repaired more quickly. One healer described how:

'I stroke the scar area for 20 minutes, warming it, and sometimes the surgery is relived, trauma comes out and the patient cries. The memory of it is no longer locked in the tissues, which relax, and scarring is reduced. This is especially important in high-tension muscles such as those of the lower back, or the neck.'

Postoperative Breathing Exercises

Many hospitals now run classes to prepare women for childbirth, and they teach breathing as the main method of reducing pain and smoothing the way out for the baby. These elementary self-care instructions prevent panic and anxiety and hasten recovery.[51] All surgical patients need them. Breathing is only occasionally to be found as part of postsurgical advice. Dr Alan Hymes, a heart surgeon at the University of Minnesota, always teaches his patients breathing exercises after surgery. He states that anxiety and pain are reduced, and there are fewer complications. When patients are asked after surgery whether they would like instructions on breathing and self-care, almost all of them say they would.[52] So where are these instructions?

Here are some basic guidelines (see also Chapter 4):

● After surgery in the chest or abdomen, coughing and strong full slow breathing will help lung function and clear out unwanted fluids.
● Hold the place of the suture as you exercise to reduce pain.
● Exercise the limbs by tensing and relaxing, rotating or lifting, unless the surgery is located there.
● Breathe with 'pacing' – slow steady regular breaths, filling the abdomen with air, and breathing out for twice as long as breathing in. This is to oxygenate the blood, start the intestines moving, and bring blood to the organs. Don't breathe too hard and fast otherwise you may get dizzy from hyperventilation. Instead let the breath 'breathe you'.
● Try the 'breath experience'. Close the eyes, breathe in through

the nose, and just be aware of the breath; where it is, where it goes, where it stops, whether it is stuck somewhere. Follow it as you breathe out. Allow yourself to feel it without controlling it, and as you do so, allow other feelings and emotions to emerge. This helps to discover and release stress and tension.

● Learn breathing techniques beforehand. Yoga teachers can teach you.

Massage and Reflexology

A skilled massage can achieve things you probably never imagined. Avi Greenberg, an experienced therapeutic masseur, explains:

'After major surgery the blood is in the trunk. I move it to the periphery by massage and reflexology. I get the energy circulating around the body again. I bring warmth to the limbs, I push the lymph channels to get them to remove the waste, to bring the blood to the area of the surgery and clean it out, to start the process of healing and prevent infections. I use ambergris and rosemary oils to warm up the muscles and improve the circulation.'

Massage is not just a pleasant way of spending an afternoon by the pool. It is a gentle and persistent method of helping healing, repairing damage and improving the flow of energy and fluids.[53] It is so obvious to use it after surgery that quite a few physiotherapists have added it to their repertoire. In the USSR physiotherapists give each patient a good relaxing massage both before and after surgery.

Reflexology is a form of massage which works on reflex points in the feet and hands in order to improve the function of organs and tissues. It is very useful in surgical patients because it does not require access to the central part of the body which may be bandaged or inaccessible. As Avi continues: 'I feel the surgical damage in the pressure points of the feet. But I do not work on the point related to the injured organ, such as the heart point after heart surgery. I work around the point, stimulating repair processes and circulation.' Reflexology is gaining acceptibility. It is used at the National Hospital for Nervous Diseases in London, especially with multiple sclerosis patients.

It is also unobtrusive: reflexologists often tell stories of surreptitious foot massages to patients in hospital, under cover of the blankets. If you have friends who know massage, you are lucky. Otherwise you can obtain a visit from a masseur by prior arrangement with your doctor. You should also request a physiotherapist trained in massage in case there is one in the hospital.

Physiotherapy

Physiotherapists are often regarded as dragons that bear down on you before you are ready and force you to move the painful parts. Others see physiotherapy as a free massage service. The truth is somewhere in between, depending on the person. Physiotherapists will see you the day after any major surgery to begin to get you on your feet again. A physiotherapist is undoubtedly an ally in your struggle to survive medical treatment. She or he will try and reduce adhesions and stiffness, and exercise your body in order to restart doped organs. If she is good she will give you self-care exercises and breathing, and she may use massage in some instances, though usually she will not have the time or the faith in it. Physiotherapists, like many medical professionals, are a bit touchy about being told what to do by the patient. If you want to request a physiotherapist ask your doctor or ward sister. It is easier to request a physiotherapist with massage training in private care.

Herbs and Essential Oils in your Surgical Survival Kit

Herb teas sweetened with honey are mild, and beneficial to add to or replace the usual hospital cuppa. Perhaps one day you will be able to order chamomile sugar-saline drips!

Four herbs can be singled out as being specially useful after surgery. For further information see Chapter 4.

● *Garlic* is one of the best anticlotting plants known and anticlotting drugs are now being made from it. It is also a great anti-infective agent. Tell your surgeon you want to take it so that he can adjust anticlotting medication accordingly.

● *Comfrey leaf and root*, in the form of tea. This plant aids healing and has unique constituents which stimulate cells to divide and repair wounds without scarring. It is also soothing to chest, throat and digestion.

● *Aromatic spices* such as ginger, cinnamon and cloves, on their own or in tea, will stimulate the movement of the intestines, warm the body, improve circulation and absorbtion of food, and prevent gas. A ginger-containing postoperative medicine called Gasex is used in India after stomach surgery.

● *Chamomile tea* prevents infection, relaxes the nervous system, and stimulates the appetite.

There are plenty of exotic medicinal plants used in various parts of the world as part of patient protection during surgical treatment. *Panax notoginseng* for example, a relative of ginseng, prevents clotting and bruising during surgery in China.

Essential oils are often used together with massage but they can be used on their own. They are the distilled aromatic constituents of various strong-smelling leaves, barks and flowers. Oils can be used for varous purposes, for example to reduce inflammation and swelling, to relax muscles, and to stimulate blood circulation on the outskirts of the body.[51]

The oils are described more fully in Chapter 4. After surgery you can use rosemary oil for self-massage to aid circulation and relax tense muscles, and wheat germ oil against inflammation. Comfrey oil or wheatgerm oil with extra vitamin E prevent scarring. When you request a massage ask for essential oils too. As the head of the London College of Aromatherapy wrote to me:

'Massage with essential oils of the chest and torso would be particularly valuable as a postoperative measure, to counteract the effects of general anaesthetic. Oils which help insomnia are also antidepressant and could be beneficial during the recovery period . . . others which are valuable in reducing scarring can be massaged over operation scars once initial healing has taken place.'

Homeopathy and Surgery

Homeopathy is a complete system of medicine. It uses minute almost invisible doses of natural remedies to create healing reactions against symptoms.[33,55] There is continuing controversy in the scientific community about homeopathy.[56] But the Royal London Homeopathic Hospital always uses homeopathic remedies to accompany surgery, particularly:

● Aconite to protect against drug effects and shock.
● Phosphorus to stop bleeding.
● Bach Flower Remedies to reduce anxiety and stress.
● Arnica for shock and tissue damage.

Homeopathic physicians claim that homeopathy will prevent repercussions of surgery on the 'vital organs and the general physical state of the patient relating to cardiac, liver and kidney function'.[57] Little attention is paid in conventional medicine to reducing the shock of surgery and anaesthesia on the organs. As Dr E. Roth of London describes it, 'I have treated patients who have had surgery and come out of the anaesthesia with severe vomiting. This is treatable more easily homeopathically than with conventional drugs. Healing after surgery is promoted with arnica or *Bellis perennis*. The surgeon will usually say that he has never seen a patient recover so quickly.'

The homeopathic physician could use any of a huge number of materials in specific cases. Professor Barriga, Professor of Surgery of the Higino Perez Hospital in Mexico, has 36 years' experience in the use of homeopathy to treat symptoms that arise from surgery. For example to help the body adjust to fluid drips and transfusions, to control clotting and bleeding, he might use Arsenicum, Alb. Ferrum Met., Pulsatilla or Millefolium. To lift confusion and depression he might use Gelsemium, Hyoscyamus Nig. or Coffea. He finds recovery is hastened by Syphilinum, Psorinum or Aluminia and there are others to strengthen heart function, to sedate and calm, to reduce nausea, pain, infections, complications and so on.[57]

As homeopathic preparations are designed specifically for a set of symptoms expressed by a particular individual, you cannot just buy them off the shelf. You can however see a homeopath beforehand for preparation for surgery, and then soon afterwards. Also Arnica and Bach Flower remedies can be purchased for self-treatment of shock and distress. You can find these remedies in a homeopathic first aid kit.

Acupuncture and Postoperative Healing: The Problem of Scarring

Scarring can be a disabling side effect of surgery, causing deep or superficial postoperative pain which can last for years. The pain clinics are full of such cases which are usually unrelieved by pain killers and require further operations and the cutting of nerves. Acupuncture help for pain in general is discussed in Chapter 5. Here we will talk about one cause – scarring – which also produces other symptoms. The scar is like a geological fault. It consists of tough fibrous tissue which heals over the surgical disconnection between body parts. It can build up tensions, strains and blockages.

Acupuncture
It is likely that the majority of patients with persistent pain, tension, insomnia and stiffness after operations could be helped by acupuncture, which treats both the visible and the deep scars. The treatment often leads to a cathartic release of tension and emotion – the earthquake that releases the strain.

For example a 47-year-old housewife came to an acupuncturist reporting severe pain in the kidney area for 12 months, along with fatigue, weakness, and loss of hearing. The woman had a history of urogenital disorders. Her last two children were delivered by Caeserean. She had had a bladder repair operation and recently a hysterecomy. Her GP, an urologist and a gynaecologist had all told her that there was nothing wrong with her and she should seek psychiatric help. When the scars were treated with acupuncture, the pattern of the pulses changed dramatically. After four scar treatments the patient described herself as feeling 30 years younger, full of energy, and resumed playing tennis.

Where recovery is incomplete and symptoms persist, go to an acupuncturist for a checkup. There are several kinds of operations where this may help a great deal, in paricular all cardiac operations and varicose vein surgery.

Other Methods

Acupuncture is an ancient system of medicine. But in today's high-tech therapy world it has spawned a number of electromagnetic therapeutic instruments. They have a more restricted field of use than acupuncture itself, but they can stimulate healing and repair. Thus if your leg is in a cast for some time, consider such treatment, on the *opposite* leg. It has been found that this can reduce wasting of the leg in plaster from about 50% to 15%. It works by rechannelling energy. Electromagnetic energy applied in the form of pulses can heal deep tissue inflammation persisting after operations.[58]

Shiatzu is acupuncture with the fingers, an Oriental massage therapy working with pressure on the acupuncture points. It is particularly suitable for postoperative patients with weak constitutions and, like massage, can be practised in hospital where an acupuncturist might not be permitted. If you know a Shiatzu practitioner consider inviting him to see you during the first few days after sugery. Shiatzu is particularly helpful after abdominal surgery which can upset the balance of the entire body. By working on points in the legs and arms, it can stimulate intestinal movement and normal organ function which is sluggish after surgery. You have to know the points so it is not suitable for self-care unless you learn it first.[59]

Which Supplements Should I Add to My Surgical Survival Kit

Food

After surgery you should get plenty of high-quality protein. Dietitians know this and will usually advise small tasty meals with concentrated protein foods. However there are also other requirements which neither the hospital kitchen nor the dietitian will provide. Their nutritional concepts are way out of date, hospital institutional cooking being notorious for preserved and processed foods, and there is little attempt, even today, to provide a diet that maximizes health and recovery. This is discussed more fully in Chapter 4.

There is a temptation today either to believe every health article and go on an indiscriminate vitamin binge in your local health shop, or alternatively to be damned with the lot of them. Here is a reasoned guide to the supplements that are important after surgery.

Vitamin C and Bioflavonoids

Vitamin C is acknowledged to help in the healing of wounds,[60] partly because it encourages the body to make collagen, the framework on which the tissues are built.[61] Surgery uses up vitamin C at a great rate and much more is needed by the white blood cells which clean up the mess and protect the body from infections.[62] Large doses of vitamin C prevent damage to joints during joint surgery.[63] Over 10 years ago the *British Medical Journal* stated that vitamin C should be given before surgery and on recovery, especially to the elderly.[64] Your hospital should give it to you. If not, request it or bring it yourself.

What the hospital will not give to you is the partner to vitamin C which helps it work, the bioflavonoids. They are citrus peel extracts which minimize the oozing of capillaries and lessen the need for transfusion during surgery.[65] Although they protect the vessels and reduce bleeding, the bioflavonoids do not interfere with the vital blood-clotting mechanism.[66] The bioflavonoids help vitamin C in collagen-building and tissue repair,[67] so make sure you get it with your vitamin C (vitamin C + bioflavonoids are commonly available in one tablet).

Zinc

Zinc is one of the minerals which you should get in your diet but often don't. Even at the best of hospitals the food has been shown to provide less than the minimum daily requirement (MDR) of 15 mg of zinc for a healthy person.[68] As a sick person, especially after surgery, you need much more, for zinc contributes to rapid wound repair[69] and also supports the immune system. It is found in mineral-rich foods such as kelp, liver and yeast or can be bought as a food supplement.

What about water?

Drink natural spring water with a high mineral content. You need the minerals, and you *don't* need the contaminants in tap water.

Vitamin E and Scar Prevention

Adele Davis stated clearly that, 'In my 37 years of working in nutrition, I have seen nothing more spectacular than the role vitamin E plays in preventing ugly scars.' After she saw 100 horrific cases of wounding and scarring (including ulcerated amputation stubs and burns) treated successfully by the vitamin E pioneers in the Shute

Clinic, London, Ontario, she started using it in her practice. For example she reports on a 7-year-old child who was operated on repeatedly for a birth defect in which the urinary passage opened at the base of the penis. 'Scar tissues had caused the urethra to become so constricted that the child screamed with pain each time he urinated, and still more surgery had to be undergone to remove scar tissue. When 200 units of Vitamin E were given daily before and after surgery the repair was successful'.[70]

Scar tissue is formed from inflammation and reduced blood supply when local blood vessels are damaged. Vitamin E increases the development of new vessels, prevents local inflammation and at the same time protects the glands and secretions necessary for recovery and repair.[71] It has been used with great success in skin grafts[72] and there is now good evidence that it prevents scars after surgery,[73] including keloids (growth on scars) that form especially on dark skin. Scars have sometimes gone years after surgery through consistently taking vitamin E.[74] The scars are helped whether they are internal or external. For example scarring after bladder surgery can cause the bladder to contract so that it can't hold very much and urination is painful. Vitamin E can reverse this.[75]

Vitamin E (tocopherol) can be taken in doses of 200–500 IU before and after surgery. Those suffering from high blood pressure should start with 100 IU and move up over a week to the chosen dose. Vitamin E in wheat germ oil should be rubbed externally on scars.

B Vitamins
The use of B vitamins is recommended for all hospital patients, mostly because of stress. Surgery exhausts the adrenal and other glands and can lead to salt imbalance, poor general functioning, exhaustion, infections and complications.[76] Supplementation of B vitamins adds greatly to patient comfort after surgery.[77] Nausea and vomiting after surgery, for example, can be prevented with vitamin B6.

Summary
The following vitamins should be part of your survival kit for surgery. They should be taken with food.

● Take the following every 4–5 hours starting a couple of days before surgery and continuing during recovery:
  500 mg vitamin C + bioflavonoids
  1 capsule kelp or alfalfa
  100 IU Vitamin E
  100 mg pantothenic acid (B5)
  5 mg B1, B2, B6

● If you are receiving sugar-saline drips, check that they are vita-minized, and if not, ask why. If you are not allowed to eat, the vitamins in the drip are especially important. In that case vitamin E capsules should be rubbed on externally as they are absorbed through the skin.

REFERENCES

1. Cochrane, A. L. *Effectiveness and Efficiency*, Nuffield Provincial Hospitals Trust, London (1972).
2. McKinlay, J. B. *Social Science and Medicine*, **13A** 541-558 (1979); US Subcommittee on Oversight and Investigations on Unnecessary Surgery (15 July 1975).
3. Schneider, R. G. *When to say No to Surgery*, Prentice Hall, Englewood Cliffs, N.J. (1982).
4. Mendelsohn, R. *Confessions of a Medical Heretic.* Contemporary Books, Chicago (1979).
5. *Drug & Therapeutics Bulletin*, **18** 7-8 (1980).
6. Galton, L. *Patient's Guide to Surgery*, Avon, N.Y. (1977).
7. Anderson, *et al*, *J. Amer. Medical Assoc.* **155** 1123 (1954).
8. Vianna, N. *et al*, *Lancet*, **1** 431 (1971).
9. Said, G. *J. of Epidemiology and Community Health*, **32** 97-101 (1978).
10. Lichter, and Pflanz, *Medical Care*, **9** 322 (1971).
11. Editorial, *The Lancet*, 1020 (3 November 1984).
12. Hodgkinson, N. *Will To Be Well*.
13. Atkins, H. *Brit. Med. J.*, **2** 423 (1972).
14. Carolyn Faulder *Breast Cancer, A Guide to Early Detection,* Pan, London (1979).
15. Editorial, *New England J. Medicine,* (2 July 1982).
16. Editorial, *Lancet*, **2** 1175 (1969).
17. Stoll, B. A. *New Aspects of Breast Cancer*, Chicago Year Book Medical Publishers (1975).
18. George, P. *British Med. J.* (July 1980).
19. Kidman, B. *A Gentle Way With Cancer,* Century, London (1983); Bishop, B. *A Time To Heal*, Severn House (1985).
20. Braunwals, E. *New England J. of Medicine,* **297** 663 (1977); Rosati, R. A. *et al*, *Postgraduate Medical Journal*, **52** 749 (1976).
21. European Coronary Surgery Study Group, *Lancet*, **1** 889 (1976).
22. Editorial, *British Medical Journal*, **1** 1163 (1979).
23. Seltzer, K. H. *Surg. Gyn Obst.* **130** 64 (1970).
24. Bainton, D. *et al*, *New England J. of Medicine*, **294** 1147 (1976).
25. Editorial, *New England J. Medicine*, 1249 (6 December 1973).
26. Mendelsohn, R. *Male Practice*, Contemporary Books Inc. Chicago (1981).
27. Bunker, J., Barnes, B. and Mosteller, F. (eds.) *Costs, Risks and Benefits of Surgery,* OUP, New York (1978).

28. Barker, M. G. *Brit. Med. J.* **2** 91-95 (1968).
29. Richards, D. H. *Lancet*, **2** 983 (1974).
30. See references 1 and 6-9.
31. Editorial, *Lancet*, (11 July 1983).
32. *Sunday Times*, March 1978. Quoted by Martin Weitz, *Health Shock*, David and Charles, London – Vermont (1980).
33. Fulder, S. *The Handbook of Complementary Medicine*, Coronet Books, London (1987).
34. Egbert, L.D. *et al*, *N. Engl. J. Med.* **270** 825-7 (1964); Healy, K. M. *Am. J. Nursing*, **68** 62-67 (1968); Schmitt, F. E. and Wooldridge, P.J. *Nursing Research*, **22** 108-116 (1973).
35. Volicer, B. J. *et al*, *J. of Human Stress,* 3-13, (June 1977).
36. Melamed, B. G. 'Psychological Preparation for Hospitalization' in Rachmann S. (ed) *Basic Readings in Medical Sociology*, Pergamon Press, Oxford (1977); Williams, J. L. *et al*, *Psychophysiology*, **12** 50-54 (1973); Reading, A. E. *Social Sci. Med.*, **13** 641-654 (1979); Sime, A. M. *J. Pers. Soc. Psychol.*, **34** 716-724 (1976).
37. George, *et al*, *J. Behav. Med.,* **3** 212-309 (1980).
38. Boore, J. R. P., *Prescription for Recovery*, Royal College of Nursing, London (1978).
39. Janis, I. L., *Psychological Stress: Psychoanalytical and Behavioural Studies of Surgical Patients*, Wiley, N.Y. (1958).
40. Kendall *et al*, *J. Consult. Clinical Psychol.*, **47** 49-58 (1979).
41. Hayward, D. J. *Information – A Prescription Against Pain*, Whitefriars Press, London (1975).
42. Wilson, J. F., *J. Behav. Medicine*, **4** 79-101 (1981).
43. Benson, H. *The Relaxation Response*, New York, Morrow (1976); Thoms, M. and Abbas, K.A., *British Medical J.*, **4** 1749 (1978); Shapiro, D. M., *Am. J. Psychiatry*, **139** 267-274 (1982); Rosa, C. *You and Autogenic Training*, New York, Dutton, (1976).
44. Langer, E. J. *et al*, *J. Exp. Soc. Psychol.*, **11** 155-165 (1975).
45. Hartsfield, J. and Clopton, J.R. *Soc. Sci. Med.*, **5** 529-533 (1985).
46. Bradley, R.A. *Psychosomatics*, **3** 1-6 (1962); Henneborn, W. J. and Logan, R. *J. Psychosomatic Research*, **19** 215-222 (1975).
47. Fredericks, L. E., *Am. J. Clinical Hypnosis*, **20** 175-183 (1978).
48. Jameson, R. M. *Brit. J. Anaesthesia*, 35 (1963).
49. Hilgard, E. R. and Hilgard, J. R. *Hypnosis in the Relief of Pain*, Kaufmann, Los Altos, California (1975); Doberneck R. C. *et al*, *Surgery*, **46** 299-304 (1959); Bouilla, K. B. *et al*, *Military Medicine*, **126** 364-370 (1961).
50. Krippner, S. and Villoldo, A., *Realms of Healing*, Celestial Art, Milbrae, California (1976); MacManaway, B. *Healing*, Thorsons's, UK, (1983); Grad. B. *Some Biological Effects of 'Laying on of Hands': A Review*, *J. Am. Soc. Psychical Research*, **59** 95-126 (1965); Magaray, C. *Med. J. Austral*, **338** 340-1 (1981).
51. Johnson, J.E. In: *Exploring Progress in Medical-Surgical Nursing Practice*, American Nurses Assoc. N.Y. (1966); Johnson, J.E., Leventhal, H. *J. Personal Soc. Psychol.*, **29** 710-18 (1974).
52. Kessler, H.W. *J. Legal Med.*, **5** 46-47 (1977).

53. Hofer, J. *Total Massage,* Grosset & Dunlap, N.Y. (1976); Kunz & Kunz *The Complete Guide to Foot Reflexology,* Thorsons, U.K. (1984); Bayly, D. *Reflexology Today,* Thorsons, U.K. (1982); Downing, G. *The Massage Book,* Random House, N.Y. (1974).

54. Price, S. *Practical Aromatherapy,* Thorsons U.K. (1983); Tisserand, R. B. *The Art of Aromatherapy,* Thorsons U.K., U.S. (1978).

55. Blackie, M.G. *The Patient, Not The Cure,* London, Unwin (1981); Smith, T. *Homeopathic Medicine,* U.K., Thorsons (1982); Vithoulkas, G., *Homeopathy, Medicine of the New Man,* New York, Arco (1981).

56. Anon., *Chemist and Drugist,* 545-551 (21 March 1981); Ruthven, M.G., *Brit. Med. J.* 1354 (19 May 1979). Gibson *et al, Brit. J. Pharmacol.,* **9** 453 (1980).

57. Barriga, J. D. 'Homeopathy and Surgery', *J. American Institute of Homeopathy,* **143** (1975).

58. Lobell, M. H. *Clinical Medicine,* **69** 8.

59. See references Chapter 4.

60. Mecray, P., *Am. J. Clin. Nutrition,* **3** 461 (1955).

61. Hamburger, *Military Medicine,* **127** 723 (1962); Pirani, C. L. *et al, Fed. Proc.* **11** 423 (1952).

62. Irvin, T. T. *et al, Surg. Gynecol. Obstet.,* **147** 49 (1978).

63. Schwartz, E. R. *et al, Laboratory Animal Science,* 683 (1981).

64. Editorial, *Brit. Med. J.,* 212 (9 February 1974).

65. Ryan, R. E. *Clinical Med.* **5** 327 (1958).

66. *Angiology,* **5** 64 (1954).

67. Harsteen, B. *Biochemical Pharmacology,* **32** 1141-8 (1983).

68. *J. American Dietetic Assoc.* (December 1976).

69. Kirschmann, J.D. *The Nutrition Almanac,* McGraw-Hill (1975).

70. Davis, A. *Let's Get Well,* Harcourt Brace Jovanovich, N.Y. (1965).

71. Matill, H. A. *Nutrition Review,* **10** 225 (1952); Roderuck, D. H. *et al, Ann. N.Y. Acad. Sci.,* **52** 156 (1949); see Harris, P. L. and other authors, in *International Congress on Vitamin E.,* (1955).

72. Edgerton, M. T. *et al, Plastic Reconstructive Surgery,* **8** 224 (1951).

73. Gibson, H. R. B. *Brit. Med. J.,* **2** 446 (1952); Blaxter, K. L. *et al, British J. Nutrition,* **6** 144 (1952); Schute, W. E. *The Complete, Updated Vitamin E Book,* Keats, New Canaan, C. T. (1975); Steinberg, C. L., *Arch. Surg.* **63** 824 (1951); Schute, E. V. *et al, J. Surg. Obst.,* **86** 1 (1948).

74. Editorial, *J. Am. Med. Assoc.,* **137** 1228 (1948); **171** 1205 (1959).

75. Van Druzen, R. E. *et al, J. Urology,* **65** 1033 (1951).

76. Howard, J. M. *Am. J. Clin. Nutrition,* **3** 456 (1955); Zucker, T. A. *Am. J. Clin. Nutrition,* **6** 65 (1958); *Nutrition Rev.,* **14** 295 (1956).

77. Leithauser, D. J. *Surg. Gynecol. Obstet.* **86** 543 (1948); Zintel, H.A. *Am. J. Clin. Nutr.,* **3** 501 (1955).

CHAPTER 7

Cancer Treatments: Chemotherapy and Radiotherapy

Chemotherapeutic drugs are very toxic. They have to be. Their effectiveness lies in the degree to which they affect cancer cells as opposed to normal cells. But because cancer cells are normal cells which have gone on a rampage, anticancer drugs damage highly active ordinary cells while attacking the cancer. The main cells affected are those in the lining of the stomach, the blood forming system and the immune system, leading on the one hand to nausea, vomiting and loss of appetite and on the other to damage to the immunity.

The nausea and vomiting are extremely distressing, occur in 90% of cases and contribute to many patients refusing treatment or at least demanding less effective dosages. They leads to 'anticipatory nausea' in about a third to a half of all patients, which occurs before the drugs are administered, or even when seeing the nurse who gives them in the local supermarket.[1] Patients lose appetite during treatment and they can't absorb vitamins and nutrients. This makes them weaker at a time when they need the strength to fight the disease. There are drugs which are given to inhibit nausea and vomiting, particularly phenothiazines (anti-psychotic drugs used in smaller doses) and recently nabilone, derived from cannabis.[2] However these drugs don't work very well, particularly against anticipatory nausea, and they have their own side effects of drowsiness and confusion.

It is one of the tragic ironies of modern cancer treatment that while attacking the cancer the treatments usually attack the body's own immune defences. Malignant tumours are continually changing and throw off seeds (metastases) which are difficult to detect and harder to treat. The patient needs every ounce of immunity during treatment, to mop up these seeds and to act against leftovers of the original tumour. Therefore by reducing the strength of immunity, chemotherapy and radiotherapy can actually promote the spread of the cancer. In a military analogy, the cancer is like a seaborne invasion beachhead pinned down by intelligent local resistance. Distant command headquarters, unfamiliar with the real conditions on the ground, call up a massive aerial bombardment of the region.

The beachhead is partly destroyed, but the resistance is also scattered, so that fresh enemy troops can rapidly drive a wedge through it and invade the countryside. This kind of thinking has lost the cancer war just as it lost the Vietnamese war.

It is an extraordinary fact that despite the wide awareness of the importance of the immunity in cancer, almost nothing is done to protect the immune system during treatment. It is sometimes possible to give drugs to suppress the immune system while the chemotherapy proceeds, so that it isn't damaged by presenting such a high profile to the chemotherapy drugs. After treatment the immunity is allowed to return to normal. This is partly successful but the immunity still takes a considerable battering.

Other side effects of chemotherapy are depression, tiredness and debility, hair falling out in about half of all cases (it regrows), occasionally ulcers and nervous-system problems with some of the drugs. The side effects depend on the type of drug and the intensity of the treatment, but in a study at the Marsden hospital about one third of patients found them unbearable, and one third dreaded them but stoically accepted them. The doctors were so alarmed about the results that they stopped the study.[3]

The end result of working against the patient's own resistance rather than with it is that battles are won but the war is lost. 60-85% of breast cancer patients will survive 5 years (depending on who's keeping the books) but only 10% will escape their cancer altogether. This is probably no more than the *real* cure rate of 100 years ago.

This means that in many cases the suffering from treatment side effects is futile with 'many, many patients being given cytotoxics that cannot possibly help them,' as Professor Timothy McElwain of the WHO advisory committee on Cancer Chemotherapy said at a meeting of the Society for Drug Research. These drugs have only been found to reliably extend life in the case of less common cancers, while the most common cancers are treated today not much more successfully than they were 40 years ago. Advances in cancer treatment very often turn out to be just wishful thinking. For example some early successes were due, it turned out, to more people surviving the operation not the cancer. Much trumpeted successes with drugs to add to surgery for breast cancer fizzled out when the figures were looked at more carefully. Short-term remissions were obtained, but at a heavy cost in side effects that didn't make it worthwhile for the patient. Long-term survival was not increased.[4] Moreover the chemicals are themselves cancer-causing agents which caused new or altered cancers to appear later on.[5]

So more conservative cancer specialists are now less willing to give the highly toxic anticancer drugs unless there is a reasonable chance that a substantial increase in lifespan will result. This can be judged by experience and certain other tests to assess the chance of the cancer spreading.

Radiation treatment kills cancer cells in the same way as the anticancer drugs. It likewise affects other normal cells that are either fast-dividing or that get in the way. The side effects of radiotherapy are very similar to those of chemotherapy, with the added problem of local burns that can occur at the point of radiotherapy. However when radiotherapy is highly focused on the particular body region involved, there could be less general sickness and loss of immunity.

There is a whole herd of sacred cows involved with cancer treatment, for example, that it is urgent, that radiation and chemotherapy are always worth doing, that patients shouldn't be told about their disease, that diet has nothing to do with cancer treatment, that the patient's psychological condition is also not relevant to the success of the treatment, and that the side effects are a necessary evil and an unfortunate part of a life-saving effort.[6] One by one these dogmas are being disproved.

The dogma which we will be concerned with is the last one. It doesn't need to be the case. There are other options to prevent the devastating side effects, but they are outside the mainstream of medicine, and so far, despite terrible patient suffering, mainstream medicine has shown little inclination to use them or even investigate them. Some years ago I wrote to a learned expert in London acquainting him with Soviet research showing that the stress of cancer surgery increases the spread of cancers, and telling him that the Soviets use certain plant drugs to prevent this spread. He wrote back a pompous letter saying that whatever went on in Vladivostok was notoriously uninteresting. Even from the limited perspective of conventional medicine this attitude is incomprehensible, because by employing these unconventional methods more patients would be able to cope with the full regimen of drugs or radiation.

The attitude arises from a concentration on the disease at the expense of the patient. The medical reaction to side effects is not to support patient health but to try to perfect the drugs or the radiation to target it more accurately on the cancer cells. In effect patient suffering from side effects has only provided another excuse to medical researchers to go off on a heroic gallop to find better weapons. Meanwhile the patient continues to be the ravaged battlefield upon which the war is waged.

Cancer Treatment Choices

The options in cancer treatment are individualistic. Oncologists (cancer specialists) begin to use new treatments before they have been fully evaluated in years-long studies. Therefore each has his personal favourite treatment combinations and all patients are involved more or less, in evaluating newer treatments. A few oncologists believe in the psychological aspect and will work with counsellors and psychologists. Others think that cancer is entirely due to random factors and patient susceptibilities are humbug. Some oncologists will be prepared automatically to give highly toxic drugs believing that the ends always justify the means. Others will not do so since they are not so convinced.

Patients have to make even more personal choices. In some cases they may not want to exchange the symptoms of cancer for the symptoms of drug effects. In other cases they may feel it's worth it to gain time. Some people are affected more by the treatments, some less. Some are more willing to fight the disease by altering their life, some are willing to let the doctors do it for them.

Because of this individuality, which is like the individuality of all disease only more visible, it is especially important that cancer patients are treated by specialists with a long experience of the disease. Treatment by doctors less familiar is often restricted to current 'formulae' for the disease. This is more likely to result in greater adverse effects for less benefit. Specialist doctors should be able to assess your progress more sensitively and on that basis decide on the most worthwhile treatments.

Information. Doctors are particularly likely to pull the wool over your eyes in relation to cancer. This is partly because they themselves find it difficult to cope with the emotional intensity of clear statements. It is partly because they need to believe in unrealistic expectations in order to keep the entire cancer-treatment machine rumbling along. Sometimes they simply don't know or they may feel that the patient doesn't want to know. Therefore they will typically downplay the disease, or lie about it to both patients and family, or worse, to the patient only, while telling the truth to everyone else. The surviving patient ought to know the truth, even if it is a devastating truth. For, if in the worst case the doctor does give the patient X months to live, the patient can at least question toxic, hopeless treatments. Moreover the patient, knowing the worst, can explore gentler ways to treat himself. Information should include that from books, self-help groups, drug literature and other previous patients, as described elsewhere in this book.

Second opinions. These are especially important as there are so many disputing views in cancer treatment, some of them absolutely the reverse of each other. For example some authorities say feed a cancer others say starve it. Generally, in a conflict between views, both of which are equally authoritative, it is usually better to choose the opinion that advises the less drastic treatment, given the current confusions.

Experimental treatments. Experimental treatments should not be refused point blank. If they are of better methods of targeting drugs, or new safer drug combinations, or immunological and unconventional methods such as hyperthermia (high temperature) treatment, they may be very helpful. But be wary of accepting treatments in which side effects are not established or those in which the benefits are questionable but irreversible damage is done to organs or immunity.

Check the statistics. Of all people who get cancer, 40% will still be alive 5 years later. This figure was more or less the same before modern treatments were developed. There are 2 million Americans living today who have lived 5 years beyond their first detection.[7] The figures tell you that some people can survive cancer with or without modern treatment. Before accepting a treatment strategy check on the survival figures for the relevant cancer, check if they have changed in the last 10 years. This will give you an independent view of how successful conventional medicine is likely to be in your case and help you to judge whether it is worth it. Check the statistics, if you can, of the department where you will be treated and compare them with the national statistics.

Be a troublemaker. Don't be timid during your treatment. It has been clearly demonstrated that those people who have a fighting, positive, active attitude to their disease are more likely to survive it, whereas those who give up hope do not survive as long. 'Those who survived the longest were real troublemakers,' said Dr Bernard Fox, Professor of Psychiatry at Boston University Medical School. 'They fought with their doctors, sought alternative opinions and methods of treatment. They refused to relinquish hope and struggled to survive.' It is now beginning to be accepted that there is no such thing as 'spontaneous regression' which is a medical admission of ignorance about cancers which disappear by themselves. The cancers tend to disappear in people who have faith, belief, emotionally uplifting experiences and active involvement in their disease.[8]

Alternative Cancer Therapies

Most of the methods discussed below to aid the side effects of conventional treatment are also used as part of alternative treatment of the cancer itself. For example hypnosis and visualization are used both as a support and as a treatment. For this reason the attitude of conventional doctors to them is a confused mixture of outrage and curiosity. On the one hand the main cancer bodies launch fierce attacks on unproven cancer therapies, and there are laws in several countries, including the UK, against alternative practitioners claiming they can treat cancer. The famous Bristol Cancer Centre had to change its name to Bristol Cancer Help Centre and when Prince Charles visited there was a storm of protest from the conventional doctors and their representatives. On the other hand there are doctors everywhere who are willing to try parts of 'unorthodox' therapies, such as hypnosis, if it can reduce pain or help patients to accept the orthodox treatment. One can only hope for a convergence of alternative and orthodox treatments in the near future so that they are both used together in a holistic manner. As a patient seeking a holistic approach there are a few things you should know.

There are no short cuts. Alternative cancer treatments are difficult, lengthy and demanding. You won't have side effects, but you will have a good deal of work – preparing juices, taking preparations and supplements, working on yourself psychologically – often on several levels at once, the dietary, psychological and medicinal. They require at the least expert guidance, and more usually a residential treatment.

The methods are traditional. They are based on self-healing and purification or detoxification. They are developments of the naturopathic view that cancers arise through dietary impurities, weak immunity, and psychological vulnerability. The cures work by eliciting the self-healing capacities of the body to remove or inactivate the cancer naturally. They use multivitamin supplements, strict dietary control, mental imagery or self-hypnosis, spiritual healing, immunological support (through herbal and organ extracts or the induction of fevers), herbs and so on. See Reference 9 for details of these methods.

Remarkable cures. Most patients arrive at alternative treatment centres when they have been pronounced incurable by doctors. The alternative practitioners claim that all these patients will have a better life and better death, that most will live longer, and that a proportion will be cured. These claims have not, as yet, been tested, although it must be said that many of the conventional cancer treatments now in use haven't been proved effective either. What can be said is that where doctors and researchers have visited these centres or tried the techniques in their practices they find patients who should be very sick apparently very well.

Treatments are not necessarily exclusive. Most patients have come to alternative cancer treatment centres after failed or unbearable medical treatment. Most also have some further medical treatment in addition to their steady progress through natural methods. One survey concluded 'Many intelligent and resourceful patients are integrating established and complementary therapies in their personal search for a treatment "program" that makes sense to them and fits their needs . . .'[10] A poll of 356 patients using complementary cancer treatments found that 40% were attracted by the natural and nontoxic aspects of complementary regimens, but only 15% rejected the conventional methods and 60% used both at the same time.[11]

Are you up to it? The methods require will, persistence and self-care. You have to take responsibility for healing yourself with the physicians as advisers. Some patients are absolutely ready for this, want to fight their disease and are frustrated at the passivity demanded by conventional treatment. Others would rather leave it to the doctor. It should also be said that dietary regimes, once begun, can give you the determination, will and energy to go through with them to the end. One woman who is now working with the Bristol Centre wanted to treat herself using natural therapies, but didn't have the strength. She went on a supervised grape juice fast for a while simply in order to develop the energy and determination to fight her cancer, which she managed to do very successfully.

Hypnosis and Imagery Can Control Side Effects

'I was having a long course of chemotherapy for leukaemia and the nausea and vomiting got worse and worse. I couldn't eat or keep a meal down when in hospital and I was sick as soon as I saw the nurse who was to give me treatments. Drugs didn't work so I called in a hypnotist. He relaxed me but I "saw through" the procedure and it didn't help. A psychotherapist was invited by my doctor, and I told him that I was sceptical but was happy for him to try.

He immediately asked me to focus on my sensations of breathing, and I let his voice come over me. He asked me to feel comfortable and relaxed and to let him know by signs how deeply relaxed I felt. I was encouraged to enjoy and revel in the feelings and then he gently woke me out of them. I don't remember very clearly what happened in my next session but I was told that after reaching a deep level of relaxation the various parts of chemotherapy treatment – travelling to hospital, meeting the nurse, receiving the injection – were described by the hypnotist with the same suggestion of comfort. I was asked to let him know by raising a finger if any of these events disturbed my comfort, and, amazingly, none of them did.

After the second session of hypnosis I didn't vomit any more and by the end of the week I was eating a full meal. The vomiting and nausea never came back.'[12]

This is a rather typical case. For the use of hypnotherapy to control the side effects of cancer treatment is a great success story. In the late 1960s and early 1970s cancer treatment centres were exploring the use of hypnosis to control pain, and researchers noticed that it also reduced or prevented certain side effects of chemotherapy and radiotherapy.[13] When they tried it with patients for whom the antivomiting drugs didn't work they invariably lost their nausea and vomiting, as well as a good deal of their anxiety. It worked with all chemotherapy agents except possibly cis-platin, the worst for the digestive system.[14]

One example is a team in Los Angeles, reporting 8 years of experience with hypnosis and psychotherapy, who first started trying to treat the cancer itself. However they drew back from this goal when they saw that the patient was often in so much distress from pain and other symptoms of both the disease and the medical treatment, that they couldn't begin to marshall the will and energy to fight the cancer itself. They found hypnosis effectively reduced pain, nausea, insomnia and anxiety, and restored appetite and energy. The patients came back to themselves so that healing could begin. 'The absolutely indispensible part of our work is the patients' experiencing the most profound quiet on a regular daily basis.' A total of 283 cancer patients had been seen, and virtually all of them had experienced a great increase in the quality of life. The survival times of those patients who already had spreading cancers (advanced metastases) of breast, bowel and lung were about three times longer than national statistics.[15]

Hypnosis cannot cure cancer. But it can lift anxiety, hopelessness, depression and discomfort so that patients gain a new positive will to fight the disease. They cease to be a victim and thus gain a new lease of life.

The climb from a depressed well of despair to a positive, living determination is as important in obtaining remissions as physical treatments. It not only gives time. It gives life. Research has confirmed that cancer patients who live longer than predicted, the 'exceptional patients', seem to be more nonconforming, independent, self-sufficient, wilful and had more insight. They could tolerate stress more easily.[16] It is probably the case that psychological strength of this kind helps the immune system attack or surround the cancer. In fact a new study at the University of Pittsburg found that cancer patients who were compliant, listless, without energy and vigour and were *resigned to their disease* had much lower cancer-attacking white cells ('natural killer' cells) than the others.

Here is a case which illustrates this. A young woman with Hodgkins Disease was receiving nitrogen mustard and her side effects were so severe that the specialists were just about to stop chemotherapy altogether. She had the added problem, quite common in such treatments, that her veins were inflamed and it was painful to inject the drug. The hypnotist induced a light trance and used a colour technique. The woman was asked to pick a colour and then to imagine flames dancing in a fireplace. The flames were all kinds of colours which eventually coalesced into the colour she chose. She was taught to imagine sinking into this colour whenever she wanted to carry out self-hypnosis. She also used the guided-fantasy approach in which she is asked to build a highly pleasant scene which she enters in order to create a sanctuary. Her particular interior sanctuary was a warm sunny morning in a mountain meadow, with all the sounds, smells, sights and impressions that go with it. She was given suggestions that the pain and inflammation, the nausea and the other symptoms would go, and they did. And as hypnosis continued she found that she could take part in life again. She travelled, completed her college degree, started some voluntary work, and could live fully during the time she had, which was longer than predicted.[17]

Childen can often enter altered states of consciousness naturally, and hypnosis is much easier than with adults. Yet children can suffer terribly from the fear, pain and discomfort of cancer treatments. It is thus essential that hypnosis or imagery is used with children receiving toxic cancer treatments. It is usually successful. For example, all children receiving cancer treatments at the Minneapolis Childrens Health Center who have unpleasant medical side effects are referred for hypnosis and imagery. The techniques used were very flexible to allow the children to suggest and develop their own themes. Of 21 children who did the exercises suggested by the hypnotist, all but two obtained substantial relief from pain and other symptoms. In one case an 8-year-old girl was under treatment for acute lymphoblastic leukaemia. She had to have painful bone marrow examinations, and was taught pain control by using 'switches' to switch off the pain at places in her body. Before the next bone marrow aspiration the therapist induced a light trance and suggested that she turn off her pain switches over the bone. The oncologist came. 'Hand-in-hand, she and the oncologist walked to the treatment room. She had no premedication. She climbed on to the table and the examination was completed in two minutes with no anaesthesia . . . she walked out with her doctor, returned to her room and, within a few minutes seemed happily engrossed in games and colouring.'[18]

Hypnosis and relaxation won't work if superficial. These methods work by unlocking powerful unconscious drives that can neutralize the effects of the anxious mind. They probably affect endorphins, brain hormones, to reduce the stress and symptoms, and these methods certainly create a shift of attention away from symptoms. Hypnosis has been found more or less equivalent to deep relaxation with guided imagery, but you must be submerged in either case. Superficial relaxation will do little more than relieve a modicum of anxiety. Nor can friendly support by a therapist or companion substitute. If the techniques are properly executed, they can be dramatic.[19]

You need homework. These are not another set of techniques done to you. You must participate by learning to do it on your own, although the hypnotist will usually aid and instruct patients in self-hypnosis, and provide a tape to help if conditions are disturbing. If you learn the technique it is available at all times. As Dr Redd, a psychologist at the University of Illinois remarked about his patients, if they vomit 'they focus on a visual point, take a deep breath and quickly slip into a quiet state of relaxation. This state continues until they fall asleep or until their 'attention' is disturbed. If interrupted or instructed to become alert, they begin vomiting immediately. Fortunately they can regain control by repeating their induction procedure.'[13]

You need expert help. Relaxation is quite easy to do by yourself, but to deal seriously with problems arising from powerful medical treatments you need expert help. The therapist ought to use those images and techniques which are personally meaningful to you. There should be no standard formulae, and no half-hearted attempts which may be worse than useless – you may feel more of a failure than you were before. Besides, the rapport established with the therapist is an important part of the process. It helps you to let go. It has been found that patients cannot use tapes properly unless they have gone through at least one, and preferably several, guidance sessions with a therapist.

Using Your Mind to Empower Cancer Treatments

Some people are destroyed by cancer treatments, others are saved by them. There are many factors which swing the balance, including personal attitude to the treatment. If you believe it will work, and encourage it, then your chances are improved.

Cancer is as much a psychological as a physical condition. The two are inseparable. This is recognized more by complementary practitioners than cancer specialists, although a few are beginning to see cancer as a 'psychobiological reaction rather than as an intrusion of a puzzling foreign matter'.[20] No cancer patient should have to go through the fruitless and heart-rending search for emotional and mental help that is usually denied them by cancer specialists:

'In a final, desperate bid for understanding I decided that all this psycho-social drama that nobody had really grasped would have to be clarified. Risking the agony of deep exposure I asked to see the doctor who seemed to have played the role of chief negotiator. He arrived, briskly pleased, imagining no doubt that I had finally come to see things his way.

"I think I know why I'm ill," I announced.

It seems funny now that I should have expected this to elicit any response other than the one I got, but I was absolutely shattered by his exasperated reply.

"Well, that doesn't make any difference to the way we treat you." '[21]

Imagery and Visualization
Imagery is well illustrated by the story of a 10-year-old haemophiliac who was bleeding profusely. The doctor began to prepare emergency measures when to her astonishment the bleeding stopped. She asked the child, 'What happened?' He said, 'Oh, I put some super-glue on it.'[22]

Imagery and hypnosis overlap a good deal. Much of hypnosis makes use of images, and people using images or visualizations are in a relaxed, semi-hypnotised state. The results of the two when measured by the crude standards of the effects on heart rate, blood circulation and anxiety are indistinguishable. Yet there are differences in practice, and here we will assess the use of imagery and visualization itself to facilitate cancer treatment.

Imagery in cancer has been made famous by the Simontons in the US.[23] It typically involves going in to visions of the cancer being attacked and cleaned up by the body's defence system. This is one of the visions: 'Your white blood cells are fish swimming in and eating up the greyish cancer cells. Project this image as if it were on a screen that you're viewing in your mind's eye. When you have that image very clear then *become* one of the fish and lead the rest of the pack into the attack. Feel yourself as the fish eating . . . at the end of each visualization, imagine yourself engaging in activities you would pursue if you were healthy. Picture yourself at the healthiest time in your life and create images of the present, feeling just that way.'

Visualizations can enhance the treatment. The chemotherapy is visualized as chemicals dismantling the tumour by not harming the cancer, the radiation machine as a friendly weapon – 'George'! This gives chemotherapy permission to do its job. Looked at that way, the side effects need not be frightening. They indicate that the drugs are working and can be accepted as an encouraging sign. The balder you are the better. For every hair that falls a cancer cell dies. It is death and then regeneration. Cancer treatment is almost like childbirth, a critical point in the interweaving of life and death.

Case Histories

Here is a case that illustrates the use of visualizations and other methods to empower treatment. It concerns Roger Parsons, who told us this story. In 1981 he developed a swollen testicle and the local hospital told him it was a teratoma. They offered him radiotherapy but instead he came down to London seeking more extensive help. He went on a nontoxic vegetarian diet and in January 1982 started chemotherapy at the Royal Marsden Hospital. At the beginning of chemotherapy he went to the Bristol Centre for advice. They instructed him in dietary measures which he pursued in the Marsden, cutting out fats, salt, sugar, meat, preservatives and caffeinated drinks; eating raw foods, grains, muesli, seeds, nuts, fruit and goat cheese. He used coffee enemas helped by nurses at the hospital.

He started relaxation and visualization with tapes. A sister at the hospital used to go with him to the Day Room and play the tapes. He fell asleep and she did the exercises! Nevertheless he felt sure it helped him relax and gain confidence. In order to remove the fear of chemotherapy he sat up all night with another patient, talking him through his fears and losing his own in the process. He agreed to chemotherapy only when he felt sure it would work. When he received the drugs 'I watched them going into my body, and I loved them, knowing they were doing me good.' He did have side effects, but they were minimal. He shaved his hair off to pre-empt it falling by itself. During the treatment he would visualise the cancer being excreted from his body every time he went to the toilet. He also spent long hours every day gazing off-centre at the sun, as he had heard somewhere that this was a support for the immune system. He took vitamins, especially vitamin C, and continued with his special diet. He said that he was glad of the hospital as it enabled him to focus exclusively on getting better.

After some months metastases in his lungs disappeared, and doctors removed the original tumour – it was 'dead', encysted, and he is cured.

Roger believes that each person must find their own mix of ways to overcome their disease and assist the treatment. But a key component is always faith and belief that they will get better. This positive, active attitude helps mop up side effects along the way. One patient who wanted to take part in her radiotherapy used to visualise the radiation as a great white healing sun that cleansed and cured her with its rays.

Another patient called Gillian, an artist, visualized the radiation as a big dragon's eye, powerful and inspiring. Gillian's chemotherapy made her frightened and withdrawn. So she sought counselling, which gave her determination which she channelled into meditation, writing and drawing, and counselling for other cancer patients in London. She had a remission for 5 years and then it recurred. This time, at Hackney Hospital she was much more prepared. She needed a mask to protect her pituitary glands from radiation damage so she decorated it beautifully, covered it with feathers and this helped her to welcome the treatment. The hospital ran visualization classes every day which she joined. She feels she has gained an extra 18 months, and lived more in this 18 months than in her life before.

A very interesting image was used by a young girl, Judy, during her radiotherapy. She imagined that her hair was like coconut matting and that each of her hairs was tied under the scalp with a little knot, so that it was impossible for them to fall out. She said that it worked.

Visualization is not easy, and, like hypnosis, it needs an experienced, trusted guide to be strong and powerful. This does not mean that the pictures have to be vivid, because it has been found that some people with less clear visualizations can be helped and others with very vivid visualizations are not. But it must involve all of you. The therapist can help by making the visualizations meaningful, relating them to your own life and personality. For example the more military attacks on cancer cells in the Simonton visualizations may have been suitable for some of their patients, but others found it too warlike and aggressive. Erica, a 60-year-old woman who has herself become a healer, felt that her cancer needed love and attention.

'The cells grow and become too big because they are seeking attention. If I give it to them they don't eat so much. I feel compassion to both my good tissues and my cancer tissues. They are both me and mine. When I had radiotherapy, I imagined myself going through my body as a garden, giving water and good things to the good plants and taking care of the weeds too.'

Problems with Visualization

The risk of visualization is that if patients do not feel they are getting anywhere they may have a discouraging sense of failure to add to others. Some of the long visualizations may turn into sleepy daydreams that meander around uselessly. The importance of a guide is to 'insert' the image into your conscious and unconscious mind. An inspiring teacher of visualization, Collette, who has been using it for 40 years in treatment, insists that this can be done with a shock. 'The image must be extremely startling to upset the patient's balance momentarily. It strikes. Then they do it intensely and briefly three or four times a day. The image actually comes from the patient, from their biography, I only induce it.' She told the story of an elderly woman with a brain tumour who couldn't move her arms. She shocked her by saying that at her age she wouldn't teach her gradually to regain movement. She would teach her flamenco! The imaginary flamenco and another visualization of cooking green peas and then eating them with a fork helped her regain a good deal of arm and wrist movement.

Like hypnosis, visualization is not a panacea. Ainslie Mears, a pioneer of the use of intensive mediation and visualization in cancer, concludes that only some 10% of patients with advanced cancer can be cured.[24] It should *always* be combined with other treatments either conventional or alternative, according to the patient's situation. Also, visualization may suit some but not others. One 39-year-old woman with metastasized breast cancer stumped the psychologist who suggested visualization: 'What? Visualization? I don't care one fig for it. I will not give one minute for my cancer.' 'Then what will you do about your anger?' replied the psychologist. 'My anger? I need every bit of it! I want it! It gives me energy. I am teaching, I am working, I am finished with my cancer!'

Healing

Spiritual healing can also be very useful in coping with and aiding treatment. Gillian went to a well-known healer after her radiotherapy had brought her a remission, in order to remove the lingering after effects of the treatment. She felt a weary tension in her body and the healing removed it completely. Healers have reported success with patients who suffer from partial paralysis due to the irradiation of a nerve during cancer treatment. The healer will focus on the nerve and help it to regenerate, in combination with both imagined and actual physiotherapy.

Three quarters of the people who come to see Matthew Manning, possibly Britain's best-known healer, have cancer, and most request help with treatment effects. He stresses that if you believe that the treatment is helpful it will be. Healing should become part of a process, so that the energy, vitality and relief given by the healer is transformed into the inner drive to be well. Healers often teach self-hypnosis to patients and encourage them to look at why they became ill. This works better if the healer and client are 'resonating' on the same wavelength, that is, they communicate well and feel good with each other. Bear this in mind when selecting a healer as with any therapist.

Diet and Food Supplements to Guard You

One of the questions that you should ask your doctor is how you should change your life style and diet so as to promote healing and enhance the treatment. Unfortunately cancer specialists, unless they work holistically, will not usually know how to answer you. 'To be unable to give a satisfactory response to this question is not only embarrassing for the physician, but it is also dangerous for the patient,' complained one cancer specialist who began to take an interest in the subject.[25]

Conventionally, a patient ought to be seen by a dietitian during cancer treatment. She will advise small appetizing high-protein meals to counter the anorexia (aversion for food) experienced by most cancer patients during treatment. She may also give certain standard vitamins such as A and D. However this is an attempt to avoid frank malnutrition rather than to assist the patient's immunity and enhance treatment.

There are several dietary approaches to cancer. They all involve the principles of completely detoxifying the body, restoring superb functioning of the organs and immunity, and adding dietary factors to expose the tumour to attack and then eliminate it from the body. The doctors who have created and administered some dietary systems see them as complete therapies in their own right which work better when the organs, blood vessels and immunity have not been damaged by chemotherapy or radiotherapy. However they also accept that many patients will want to receive conventional treatments, and encourage these dietary approaches as partners to reduce symptoms, improve the quality and length of life, and prevent the side effects of treatment. We will look at two dietary systems which are showing good results: the naturopathic, for example the therapies pioneered by Hans Moolenburgh and Max Gerson, and the macrobiotic.

The Naturopathic Diet (The Gerson Diet)
This is a highly detailed and organized system, more or less a full-time job, which is described in Reference 9. The main components are as follows:

● No sugar, fats, alcohol, coffee, tea, tobacco, food preservatives or additives and almost no salt. This eliminates the stress of further contamination of the body.

● High-fibre vegetarian diet with added liver extract. The vegetables should be young, fresh and biologically grown on good soil. About 20% of the diet should be raw vegetables especially carrots, radish, sprouts, beets, greens, cucumber, parsley, onions and dandelion tops. Cooked vegetables should be minimally cooked or steamed, in stainless steel or enamel saucepans.

● Only cold-pressed oils, especially sesame or olive oil.

● Minimal starches, depending on the condition of the patient, derived from seeds, oatmeal or muesli and brown rice.

● Protein-rich seeds such as pulses, sesame, buckwheat, all nuts, pumpkin and sunflower seeds, mung beans, and apricot kernels (which are therapeutic).

● Spring or mineral water. No chlorinated, fluoridated or recycled water.

● Fruit. Dried or fresh.

● Vegetables and fruit should also be prepared in the form of total juices, at least 1 litre/2 pints per day.

● Garlic. Kelp. Yeast.

● Raw milk products, particularly yoghurt and kefir, at certain stages of the treatment only.

● A number of organ extracts and nutritional supplements.

It is essential that this diet is supervised and properly designed for each patient, and it should be combined with other procedures such as enemas, purges, herbal medicines, fasts, exercise, and psychotherapeutic or meditative work. The entire system can be obtained at residential or day centres in the US, UK and Europe.

The Macrobiotic Diet

This is a purifying dietary system based on Oriental concepts of harmony and balance. It too must be continually altered depending on a patient's progress through the disease, and therefore needs to be supervised by an expert. It is not as specifically designed to cure as the naturopathic cancer therapies and therefore needs to be combined with other treatments.

It involves balancing pure natural foods, particularly brown rice, fresh specially prepared vegetables, dried pulses and beans, seaweeds, buckwheat and Japanese soya products such as miso, according to the constitution and condition of each person. It holds to the prohibitions of sugar, alcohol, etc. described above, but does not add all the special food factors and supplements found in the Gerson diet.

Leaving aside the question of remissions, there are a great many cases, mostly unpublished, where the diets have helped to prevent destructive effects of cancer treatments. A study in 1966 with 56 patients found that 9 out of 10 of those given an enriched natural diet with their irradiation improved, compared with 5 out of 10 of those who did not receive the diet.[25] The only published research trial of the Gerson diet is that still in progress under Dr Peter Lechner at the largest hospital in Austria, the Landeskrankenhaus. He was so impressed with the apparent health of patients with advanced cancer whom he saw at the Gerson Centre in Mexico that he set up a trial in which one group of 40 patients were given the diet together with conventional treatments, and compared with other patients who were given conventional treatments alone. All the patients had advanced cancers of the digestive system which had spread elsewhere. He reports that his diet patients were in excellent general condition even in very advanced cases, and were surviving much longer than all predictions. He was mostly able to replace narcotics with aspirin-type painkillers. None of the patients needed tranquillizers, sedatives or similar drugs, and he reports that not one of the diet patients needed to have their chemo- and radiotherapy reduced because of side effects. These patients 'were protected against depressed blood counts, loss of hair, depressed liver function, and other well known negative side effects of chemotherapy.'[26]

We talked to Diana, a small, determined and strong-willed 46-year-old woman who first noticed a lump on her breast in September 1981, which was not diagnosed as cancer until 1984, by which time it had ulcerated and spread. She underwent six weeks of intensive radiotherapy even though the radiotherapist felt it might be too late, and was given six months to live. She started a strict, guided macrobiotic diet at the same time. She didn't feel sick or tired throughout the treatment which she was told was exceptional. After radiotherapy the breast healed completely. The radiotherapist was very pleased and said that 'He had seen it happen once before'. She refused surgery and concentrated on her diet, with her sister cooking it, and going on it herself to encourage her. Though she lost a lot of weight, which worried the doctors, she felt she was getting better, and managed a second course of radiotherapy without any side effects other than superficial burns. She is not through the wood yet, but at present has no detectable metastases. She looks well, with bright eyes and an enthusiastic lively presence.

Vitamins and Dietary Supplements

Vitamins and supplements should, for best results, be part of a programme to examine and renovate all parts of your life style from the water and air you take in to the activities of your daily life. However there are important benefits to be had by taking the right vitamins during cancer treatment. The protective effect of vitamins has already been discussed in relation to diagnostic X-rays. Since radiotherapy may use doses 1000 times greater, the need for vitamins is correspondingly more profound. Both radiotherapy and chemotherapy drastically deplete the body of vitamins, which should be made up.

Vitamin C

Professor Linus Pauling, Nobel Laureate and one of the greatest scientific figures of our time, shocked the medical world by announcing that vitamin C treatment can prolong the lifetime of cancer patients, alleviate their suffering and help in the side effects of treatments.[27] We have come a long way in the 10 years since then, and know much more about nontoxic metabolic and nutritional treatments. The original reports announced that 100 patients in the Vale of Leven Hospital in Loch Lomonside, Scotland, treated under the supervision of Dr Ewan Cameron, survived four times as long as 1000 similar patients, if they were given vitamin C. This was hotly denied by further careful clinical research in the US which couldn't find any prolongation of life with vitamin C.[28] Sniping continues, but the current view is that vitamin C, though not a cancer cure, can help people to tolerate chemotherapy and radiotherapy. Studies have shown that when vitamin C was combined with the cancer-killing drugs methotrexate or 5-FU they were more effective in attacking cancer cells.[29]

Scientists at Wake Forest University found that monkeys given vinblastine and vincristine, anticancer drugs from the vinca plant, avoided weight loss or hair loss when they were given vitamin C, without losing the positive effects of the treatment. Linus Pauling concludes, 'There is some evidence that cancer patients undergoing radiotherapy have an increased requirement for ascorbic acid (vitamin C) and that satisfying this increased requirement protects against some of the harmful effects of irradiation as well as potentiating the therapeutic response.'[30]

Vitamin C is probably fulfilling several functions. It is an 'antioxidant,' that is, a substance which protects against free radical damage, the main damage caused by radiation. This is discussed more fully in Chapter 3. It also helps to neutralize toxins produced during treatments, protect and enhance the immune system, and support the adrenal and other glands in coping with the immense stress imposed by such drastic treatments. Vitamin C, like other vitamins, should not be taken in very large doses, above 10 gm per day, without advice from a nutritional expert or holistic doctor. It can have side effects of its own during cancer treatment.

Vitamin E and Other Antioxidants

Other antioxidants would, according to this reasoning, also be effective, and vitamin E has been shown to enhance the effect of vincristine on tumours and prevent damage to heart, skin and lungs produced by adriamycin and bleomycin.[31] A combination of E and C has been used to protect against various side effects of radiotherapy, with some success.[32] Other antioxidants that may be useful, because they work as a team with vitamin C, are selenium, cysteine and glutathione (see Chapter 3).

B Vitamins

The B vitamins aid the liver to remove the toxins created during treatment. They, together with vitamins A and C, also prevent damage to the immune system so as to help remove dead cells and prevent the cancer spreading. These vitamins can prevent the tiredness and debility that result from cancer treatments.

A study some years ago at the Montefiore Hospital in New York compared patients who received intensive radiotherapy with and without yeast supplements. Those who took 3 tablespoons of yeast starting a week before experienced far fewer side effects.[33] The most important vitamin to protect against nausea and vomiting is B6, but pantothenic acid and folic acid are both useful in preventing toxicity.

Vitamin Dosages

A high-dose vitamin regimen should be taken at least one week before the start of radiotherapy or chemotherapy. It is very hard to give an absolute dosage guide because it varies from person to person depending on the state of the liver, body weight, condition of the disease and so on. Therefore it is important to seek the advice of a holistically-minded doctor who will guide you. Indeed this is one way in which you can involve your own practitioner in your general care without interfering with the treatment itself.

A complex mixture of supplements is now being tested by the Peninsula Hospital, Far Rockaway, New York, in a well-organized clinical trial, as an aid to patients during chemotherapy and radiotherapy. It consists of a daily dosage of:

(Vit E)	– dl-Alpha tocopherol	600 IU
('DMG')	– Dimethyl glycine	120 mg
(Vit B6)	– Pyridoxal phosphate	18 mg
(Selenium)	– Sodium selenite	225 microgm
(Vit B3)	– Niacinamide	150 mg
	Glutathione	150 mg
(Vit B2)	– Riboflavin-5-phosphate	75 mg
(Vit B1)	– Thiamine HCl	75 mg
	Calcium pantothenate	66 mg
(Vit C)	– Ascorbic Acid	180 mg
	L-cysteine	300 mg
	Zinc sulphate	45 mg
(Vit A)	– Beta carotene	30,000 IU

The above mixture gives an idea concerning required dosages. A simpler mix of supplements is given in Chapter 3, page 33. Note that B complex vitamins should be taken together, and a good diet, as defined in Chapter 4, should be combined with the supplementation programme. Check with your doctor if there are any special nutritional requirements associated with the particular chemotherapeutic drug he is giving you. For example cis-platin has been shown to deplete zinc and magnesium because of its effects on the kidneys, and methotrexate prevents calcium and magnesium from being absorbed from food.

Radiation Burns and Hair Loss

Excellent results have been obtained with vitamin E to prevent radiation burns, a frequent and very unpleasant side effect of radiotherapy. The usual problem is that the burns are not given a chance to heal because of repeated radiation treatment. Vitamin E prevents the burning in the first place, and greatly diminishes the pain and subsequent scarring of the area.[34] Vitamin E in wheat germ oil should be applied liberally to the area before and after every treatment and once or twice a day in the interval. If it is available only in capsules pierce them with a pin and apply the contents.

Aloe vera gel is probably the best material for the cure of radiation burns once they are there. Japanese survivors of the atomic bombs who applied *Aloe vera* gel to radiation burns healed more rapidly and with less scarring than those that did not. There is relief from pain and inflammation, and more rapid regrowth of tissues. *Aloe* can dry the skin so other skin care agents should be added. A 55-year-old woman from Oxford had a mastectomy followed by eight weeks of radiation treatment twice a week. She was in considerable pain from the burns which didn't heal. A friend of mine gave her little pots of *Aloe vera* plants to have at home. Morning and evening she would break a leaf and apply the juice. From the very first day, she said, the pain was reduced, the skin looked better and she was able to give up painkillers.

Preventing Hair Loss
The American International Hospital in Illinois has found that an 'ice bonnet' placed on the scalp 15 minutes before chemotherapy and radiotherapy and left on 30 minutes afterwards, will prevent at least half of all patients losing their hair. However the hair does grow back, sometimes quite luxuriantly, if it falls out during cancer treatment.

Shingles and Viral Diseases

The inhibition of immunity caused by cancer treatments leaves the patient extremely vulnerable to infections during the period of treatment. Usually patients are given gamma-globulin injections to improve resistance, and any onset of an infection is quickly treated by antibiotics. But shingles and viral infection can occur at this time, and there is little that is conventionally available apart from painkillers to deal with these. I have seen how excruciating shingles can be, as a relative had it for three months as a result of cancer treatment.

At the onset of a virus infection increase the dose of vitamin C to 2-5 gm per day. Find a source of L-lysine, an amino acid which is helpful in diminishing virus multiplication. This may be available through holistic practitioners who should be consulted. Vitamin E oil, as described in the last section, is quite effective when rubbed over the shingles. Also take vitamin E capsules internally as described above. Acupuncture and TENS treatment (See Chapter 6) can be used to dull the pain of nerve inflammations.

Herbal and Homeopathic Remedies Against Treatment Symptoms

Where there is an existing herbal tradition it would be unthinkable to allow people to go through the devastating experience of cancer treatment without calling on the rich resource of plant medicines to help them. In Switzerland many family doctors will automatically send cancer patients to a phytotherapist for herbal treatment of chemotherapy symptoms such as poor appetite, tiredness, nausea, vomiting, skin irritations and liver upset. There is no single prescription for these side effects – different herbalists will prescribe different herbs depending on their experience and the particular symptoms involved. The symptomatic use of herbs is ancient, well tried, and often remarkably successful. Some particularly useful materials are:

Aloe vera. This is an important part of natural cancer treatment, taken internally in prescribed amounts. It can protect the intestines and restore their function if they are affected by chemotherapy and radiotherapy. It provides curative rather than symptomatic treatment. Like many bitter/aromatic herbs, it also stimulates the appetite and digestion. *Aloe vera* can be combined with classical bitter herbs such as angelica root or rhubarb and these 'bitters' are available from herbal suppliers. Alternatively you can take *Aloe vera* by itself as a juice or in capsules.

Alginates and seaweed products. Alginate, a mucous material extracted from seaweeds, is now used as part of standard protection against radioactivity. It has been shown that a similar type of extract of the seaweed *Digenea simplex* prevented nausea, loss of appetite, debility, and some pain, when given to 162 patients after irradiation for metastasized bone cancer.[35] Add seaweed products, including jellies or cooked food containing agar-agar, to your diet.

Icelandic moss/Irish moss. These are the classical Western herbs, along with slippery elm bark, which protect the digestive system by soothing it with a mucilaginous coating. They are very similar to seaweed extract in action, and may be more widely available.

Marijuana and cannabis. It has been discovered that this herb, the archetypal 'weed', is effective at reducing the nausea and vomiting arising from chemotherapy. The National Cancer Institute is making Δ-THC, the active ingredient, available to researchers, and many cancer patients have taken it during chemotherapy with considerable success. In the last few years a half-dozen synthetic drugs have been developed, based on the cannabis components,[36] and one, nabilone, is in general use. It seems absurd that the herb cannabis, which is cheap, natural, safe and well tried, is illegal so that not even doctors can prescribe it without permission, whereas its main ingredient chemical, requiring tens of millions of dollars to develop, and with known and unknown side effects, is described as a welcome discovery.

I haven't received any direct reports of the use of cannabis along with chemotherapy. However it is an option to consider. It should be eaten rather than smoked. The euphoria may be desirable to some and not to others, but if you welcome it and accept it, it too can help you.

Herb teas. The best are chamomile, cinnamon, ginger and black horehound to prevent nausea and vomiting. Take them frequently.

Homeopathic remedies. These can be used to deal with specific symptoms as they occur. But they must be prescribed by a homeopath after the proper in-depth diagnostic symptom picture is established. You cannot prescribe them for yourself. Homeopathic remedies against unwanted symptoms are based on the materials that create the same symptoms in the healthy. For this reason homeopaths have used highly diluted preparations of radium bromide, uranium nitrate or cadmium sulphate against radiation sickness, and phosphorus or fluoric acid to help cure radiation burns. I received a letter from a woman in Wales who had had 25 radiation treatments. After the eighteenth the doctors had to halt treatment because her sensitive skin suffered from burns. A homeopath gave her *cantharis* six times a day. A week later she went for the rest of her treatments which were so successful that the nurse remarked about her tough skin, and the radiotherapist said he had never known such healing.

How to Protect Your Immunity During Treatment

The hidden side effects of radiotherapy and chemotherapy may be more serious than the obvious ones, particularly the fact that it weakens vitality and the immune system. The same chemotherapeutic drugs are, in fact, used conventionally to suppress the immunity in the rare cases (eg organ transplants) when this is required. The cancers are there because the patients have a hole in their defences in the first place, for environmental, psychological or constitutional reasons. So further loss of immunity can be disastrous; it can allow the cancer to spread and new ones to grow. There is evidence that even the stress of surgery or biopsy encourages the spread of cancer cells. A 7-year study in Germany found that women who had biopsies tended to have metastases sooner than women who did not.[37] The end result is as I have already said: treatment wins the battles but loses the war.

Oriental medicine has developed immune-supporting remedies just as Western medicine has developed immune-destroying ones. Cancer treatment in Oriental medicine mainly consists of supporting patient vitality and directing the body's intelligent resistance to deal with the cancer. There are also milder anticancer drugs now used, developed from plants, which do work against cancers but not in such a blunderbuss fashion as Western drugs. For example the Chinese use starch-like compounds from the plant *Polyporus umbellatus* to stimulate the immunity against cancer, while the plant drugs indirubin, curcumol, harringtonine, monocrotaline, and sophocarpine are all used in China as anticancer agents.[38] Chinese medicine can offer protection of the immunity and vitality during chemotherapy and radiotherapy unmatched by any Western remedy, with the possible exception of mistletoe. The best available remedies are as follows.

Astragalus, Ligusticum and Codonopsis. These are three of the main specific immune-stimulating herbs of Chinese medicine. They are not generally available but can be found with the help of a herbalist. They should be used only with expert guidance. At the Cancer Institute in Peking these herbs were given to patients with advanced liver and lung cancer, along with radiation and chemotherapy. The herbs protected the functions of the glands, improved the production of blood, and increased survival from 30% to 70% over one year. Astragalus and Ligusticum have been investigated at the National Cancer Institute and at other centres in the US with nearly 600 cancer patients. They have found that these herbs restored function in the immune system in 90% of cancer patients. The patients recovered more quickly from chemotherapy or radiotherapy and lived longer. They didn't suffer from as much depression of the bone marrow, or digestive disturbances. These herbs are difficult to find in Europe, except in the Chinese community, but are sold in the US. They should not be taken as potential cancer cures, but as aids to treatment, and they should always be taken with a professional herbalist's or acupuncturist's advice.

Eleutherococcus. Russian research has found that when animals with cancer underwent an abdominal operation the percentage of animals whose cancer spread increased from 49% to 78%. If they were given the Far Eastern herb *Eleutherococcus senticosus* (Siberian ginseng) there was no increase in metastasis as a result of the operation,[39] and for this reason animals survived longer.

Among many Soviet studies is one at the Petrov Oncological Institute in Leningrad. There 5 gm of *eleutherococcus* or a look-alike placebo were given every day to 107 patients receiving surgery and chemotherapy for stomach cancer, and the herb or placebo were continued for a year afterwards. Patients given the *eleutherococcus* were able to tolerate 50% more anticancer drugs, they felt better during treatment, and their average lifespan was increased from 12 to 17 months. These studies have resulted in the Soviets using *eleutherococcus* widely to improve the resistance of patients to cancer treatment.

The Chinese are working to extract an immune-supporting material from *eleutherococcus* which they call *ciwuja*. Although *eleutherococcus* is unlikely to be as strong an immune protective as the Chinese herbs described above, it may have additional benefits to vitality and general wellbeing. This is also the case with ginseng. *Eleutherococcus* can be bought in Europe and should be taken at a high dose (5 gm per day). It is completely nontoxic.

Ginseng is well known for its ability to help cope with stress. This includes the stresses of chemotherapy and radiotherapy. Professor Brekhman of the USSR Academy of Sciences, the imaginative father figure of research into the Oriental 'adaptogenic' remedies, found that he could double the survival of irradiated animals by feeding them ginseng or *eleutherococcus*. During the last few years a team of scientists led by Dr Yonezawa of Osaka Prefecture Radiation Centre have investigated how ginseng does this, concluding that it is because it gives a sharp boost to the blood factories of the body, so that they quickly restore the protective white cells and other blood components. The radiation doses used in these studies were higher than patients receive. However I have had several reports from people who described how ginseng has helped them with tiredness, illness and debility during cancer treatment, and for these purposes ginseng appears to be uniquely effect. For advice on taking ginseng see Chapter 4.

Acupuncture. A client of my own acupuncturist told me:

'I had chemotherapy two weeks in every month for six months, and acupuncture after each two-week period. After chemotherapy treatment I would always plummet right down; acupuncture did delay plummeting but did not avoid it totally . . . I now feel that I should have had it straight after the injections and it might have helped more . . . after radiotherapy I felt totally washed out. I had no strength or energy and could hardly get out of a chair . . . Acupuncture was the only treatment that kept me going. It gave me energy and I could get around.'

This was a young research chemist with Hodgkins Disease. Acupuncture can help with the generally low level of vitality and energy experienced during cancer treatment. Research in China has shown that it can also help protect the blood-forming and immune tissues during radiotherapy, and can aid with symptoms, particularly insomnia and nausea.[42]

Acupuncture in such a situation is a daunting challenge to the acupuncturist. He should be a competent traditional acupuncturist who treats organ systems, not just pain. For he must be able to support internal functions, such as immunity, damaged by cancer treatment, otherwise the main advantage of acupuncture would be missed.

Shiatzu can help similarly, though to a lesser extent, but all massage treatments in cancer patients must be done by an expert and never directly around the tumour, in case they spread it. One Shiatzu practitioner wrote that 'following radiotherapy, chemotherapy and surgery the patient's energy (Ki) was very depleted. Using Shiatzu seemed to bring her back to life'.

Mistletoe (*Viscum album*). The use of preparations containing this plant in cancer has an old tradition in Europe. The plant is recognized by Rudolf Steiner's anthroposophical movement, a Swiss-based humanistic/mystical movement, to have potential cancer-healing properties, and this has been borne out by subsequent research.[43]

The plant has similar starchy materials to some of the Oriental remedies described above, and acts as an immune stimulant. For this reason its use just before and during conventional cancer treatments can help prevent spreading of the cancer.[44] In several hospital studies mistletoe preparations have increased survival well above predictions, and it has helped patients to recover energy, health and appetite.[45] Like the other remedies it should be used with the advice of a herbalist.

Note: Make sure that the thymus gland at the base of the throat is shielded during radiotherapy. It is one of the key components in your immunity, and is often not considered by radiotherapists.

REFERENCES

1. Whitehead, V. M. *New Eng., J. Med.,* **283** 199-200 (1975).
2. Chang, A. E. *et al, Annals Int. Med.,* **91** 819-824 (1979).
3. Palmer, V., *et al, British Medical J.,* **281** 1594-7 (1980).
4. Brinklely, D. *British Medical J.,* **288** 1709-10 (1984), Le Fanu, D., *The Health Services (4 November 1983).*
5. *Whitehouse, J. M. A. British Medical J.,* **290** 261-2 (1985).
6. Angell, *World Medicine,* **26** (18 October 1978); Cairns, J. *Cancer, Science and Society,* San Francisco (1978).
7. American Cancer Society, *Cancer Facts and Figures,* Annual Reports (1982).
8. Stoll, B. (ed.) *The Mind and Cancer Prognosis,* London (1979); Meares, A. *Lancet,* **978** (5 May 1979).
9. Gerson, M. *A Cancer Therapy – Results of 50 Cases,* Totality Books; Bishop, B. *A Time to Heal,* Severn House, London (1985); Pearce, I. *The Gate of Healing,* Neville Spearman, Jersey; Rohe, F. *Metabolic Ecology,* Wedgstone, Kansas (1982).
10. Lerner, M. *Advances,* **2** 31-43 (1985).
11. Cassileth, B. R. *et al, Annals Int. Med.,* **101** 105-112 (1984).
12. Abstracted from Hoffman, M. L. *Am. J. Clinical Hypnosis,* **25** 173-176 (1983).
13. Redd, W. M. *et al, Am. J. Clinical Hypnosis,* **25** 161-172 (1983); Zeltzer, *et al, J. Paediatrics,* **97** 132-138 (1980).
14. Conway, A. V. *Holistic Medicine,* **1** 43-55 (1986).
15. Newton, B. *Am. J. Clinical Hypnosis,* **25** 104-113.
16. Achterberg, J., et al, *Psychotherapy Theory, Research and Practice,* **14** 416-422 (1977).
17. Dempster, C. R. *et al, Int. J. Clinical Exp. Hypnosis,* **24** 1-9 (1976).
18. Olness, K. *Am. J. Paediatric Hematol./Oncol.,* **3** 313-321 (1981).
19. Lyles, J. N. *et al, J. Consulting Clin. Psychology,* **50** 509-524 (1982); Burish, T. G. *et al, Oncol. Nursing Forum,* **10** 32-35 (1983).
20. Bahnson, C. B. and Bahnson, M. B. *Annals, N. Y. Acad. Sci.,* **125** 827-845 (1966).

21. Brohn, P. *Gentle Giants*, Century Hutchinson, London (1986).
22. Ament, P. *J. Medicine*, **13** 233-240 (1982).
23. Simonton, O. C. *et al, Getting Well Again*, Bantam, N.Y. (1980).
24. Meares, A. *Austral. Fam. Physician*, **9** 322 (1980).
25. Berkeley, G. E. *Cancer: How to Prevent It and How to Help Your Doctor Fight it*, N.J., Prentice Hall.
26. Lechner, P. Paper read at Congress of Austrian Surgeons, Graz, Austria (21 June 1984); *J. Alt. Med.*, 8 (October 1985).
27. Cameron, E. and Pauling, L. *Vitamin C and Cancer*, Warner, N.Y. (1977); Cameron, E. and Pauling, L. *Proc. Nat. Acad. Sci. USA*, **73** 3685-9 (1976).
28. Moertel, C. G. *New Eng. J. Med.*, **312** 137-141 (1985).
29. Prasad, K. N. *et al, Proc. Nat. Acad. Sci., USA*, **76** 829-832 (1979).
30. In: Challen, J. and Lewin, R. *Let's Live*, 30 (May 1985).
31. *Medical Tribune* (31 March 1982).
32. Sokoloff, B. *et al, J. Clinical Investigation*, **30** 395 (1951); Field, J. B., *et al, Am. J. Med. Sci.*, **1** 218 (1949).
33. Samachson, J. *et al, Arch. Biochem. Biophys.*, **88** 355 (1960).
34. Schute, E. V., *Annals. N.Y. Acad. Sci.*, **52** 358 (1949); Black, M. I. *Clinical Med.*, **57** 112 (1950).
35. Claudio, F. and Standardo, B. *Proc. Int. Seaweed Symposium*, **5** 369 (1965).
36. Razdan, R. K. and Howes, J. F. *Medicinal Research Reviews*, **3** 119-146 (1983).
37. Quoted in Rohe, F. ref. 9. See also Chapter 6 ref. 17.
38. Peigen, X., *J. Ethnopharmacology*, **7** 95-109 (1983).
39. Yaremenko, K. V. *Mater. Izuch. Zhenskenya Drugiskh Lek. Sred. Dal'n. Vostoka*, **1** 109-116 (1966); Stukov, A. N. *Problems of Oncology*, **12** 57-60 (1966); ibid **13** 94-95 (1967) (in Russian).
40. Brekhman, I. I., *et al, Meditisne Radiologia*, **5** 33-36 (1960) (in Russian).
41. Yonezawa, M. *et al, J. Radiat. Res.*, **26** 436 (1985).
42. Yuqing, X. *et al, Chinese Acup. and Mox.*, **4** 6-8 (1984).
43. Bloksma, N. *et al, Immunobiol.*, **156** 309-319 (1979); Anderson, L. A. *Pharmaceutical J.*, 437-439 (16 October 1982).
44. Evans, M. R. and Reece, A. W. *Bristol Medico-Chirurgical J.*, **88** (1974); Nienhaus, J., *et al, Experientia*, **26(5)** (1969).
45. Salzer, G. *Onkologie*, **1** 264-267 (1978); ibid. *Zeitschrift fr. Allgemeinmedizin*, **5** s. 20-23 (1981).

CHAPTER 8

Preventing Infections in Hospital

Risks of Receiving an Infection in Hospital

The shiny vinyl flooring, the pervasive smell of germicides and disinfectants, the crisp white coats, all give an impression that hospitals are clean sterile places, certainly more than your dusty front room with its dog scratching in front of the fireplace. The reverse is true: hospitals are a zoo of exotic germs. There may be fewer per square centimetre than on your living room carpet but they are far more deadly.

One in 10 people admitted to hospital catch an infection there that they didn't have before. In the US 100,000 people die from these hospital infections every year, and according to some authorities it may be more. Professor Schimpff, of the University of Maryland School of Medicine, suggested that 137,500 people die from pneumonia caught in US hospitals every year. In fact these hospital-born infections (HBI) led to the discovery of the existence of germs in the first place. The Viennese doctor Ignatius Semmelweiss noticed in 1848 that women whose babies were delivered by medical students died from fevers three times more often than women delivered by midwives. He realized it was contamination but when he tried to get doctors to wash their hands he was hounded so much that he ended up in an asylum.

The fact is that all kinds of diseased fluids, faecal matter, discarded tissues, rubbish, food, nappies, catheters etc. are collected by people who go in and out of wards; that beds, stethoscopes, hospital equipment, lavatories and washbasins are in intimate contact with patient after patient, and that air conditioning and heating stir up and blow in dust and germs all over the place.

Recent hospital outbreaks of Legionnaires Disease, a very unusual and fatal infection, were traced to the alien germs hiding in the air conditioning systems. The hospital is the breeding ground of completely new and dangerous organisms. The most frightening to doctors is a new strain of the common-or-garden staphylococcus called MSRA, dubbed by the media as super-staph, which is resistant to virtually all the available antibiotics. It has been identified in hospitals all over England and has led to wards and Intensive Care Units being closed. 'It has caused deaths in people who were basically well before they came into hospital. They have had an operation and died from an infection', stated the head of a group of doctors trying to find a way to stop it.[2]

Deaths are less common than long and sometimes disabling illnesses that come from such infections. Most people who enter hospital are blissfully ignorant of the potential risks. Here is a case with rather exteme consequences. 'In March 1976, I went to see the consultant for a hip operation, for which I was sent to hospital. I had the operation done in which I caught something in the theatre. I got a bug in the blood stream which put paid to me. I never knew what this would lead to. I was in and out of hospital like a yo-yo, having various operations on my left leg . . . I was on crutches for nearly 2 years until the strength of my left leg gave way and I collapsed to the floor. I then 'phoned the consultant and saw him. He saw my hip and I said "It's still weeping". He turned around and told me to have it off, in a hard sort of way. He said come back and see me when you have made your mind up.

'To cut the story short, the leg was no use so I had it amputated. The whole of the left leg. This was the result of catching a bug . . . now I am a wheelchair victim. I could tell you lots more but it would take too long.'[3]

Why does this happen? After all, hospitals are supposed to be the Mecca of sterility. There are several reasons for it. The first is ignorance. It turns out that all the swabbing, sterilizing and disinfecting may sometimes be worse than useless. An official at the Central Public Health Laboratory in the UK told me confidentially that slopping things with disinfectant was like expelling ghosts. Their tests had shown that it spread germs. Tests had also shown that the slippery vinyl floors did not give out less germs than carpets, that clean personal nightgowns had no more germs than hospital gowns, and that visitors made no difference to the level of germs. Yet these are rituals that seriously inconvenience patients. On the other hand certain procedures which are recommended by the authorities are not done. These include washing of hands after touching patients, and not having standing water in sinks and other places.

Besides, the more dangerous germs that lurk in hospitals rather than the hearth are encouraged by modern medicine itself. Antibiotics have been used so widely that the germs, being apparently wiser than human beings, are winning the battle and evolving into dangerous new resistant strains such as MSRA. The common use of wide-spectrum antibiotics, and antibiotics in farming, could put medicine back 50 years to the days when a minor infection could be lethal.

There is another reason which concerns us here more directly. It is that patients in hospital are often so weak and vulnerable that they catch infections even from the germs that normally live on the outside of their body as harmlessly as ants in the grass. Medical specialists, of course, cite this as their main excuse for the high rate of infections. But it is not at all as good an excuse as it sounds. For a good deal of the weakness and vulnerability comes from the hospital milieu itself. After all, you don't need to worry about getting pneumonia along with treatment by an acupuncturist or homeopath.

It is not that hospital doctors want to lower resistance, they simply don't understand how to raise it. The philosophy and practice of modern medicine, as it is taught in medical schools, is to look for specific causes of disease and attack them wherever they can be found. So doctors chase after germs like angry farmers shooting at birds. The birds escape to another farm and the crops are trampled in the process.

The task of this chapter, clearly, is to advise on ways to improve your resistance while under medical treatment. It will look more carefully at how the damage to your resistance happens and how to protect yourself against it, and then how to increase your natural immunity.

How Immunity is Lowered in Hospital

The immune system is a flexible defensive system, capable of reacting to all kinds of alien agents which threaten the body, from viruses to bacteria, from smoke particles in smokers' lungs to the mutated cancer cells that may crop up in their bodies. It consists, broadly, of protective proteins which circulate in the blood, and different kinds of white cells which are made in the thymus gland and spleen and distributed everywhere, especially in the lymph. The immune system acts by testing the mettle of the visitor, memorizing its characteristics, running off to clone weaponry specifically designed to attack the invader and then mounting a concerted assault.

Researchers have found that grief reduces the ability of the immune system to mount defences against infections, germs or stray cancer cells. A man is ten times more likely to be ill in the year after his wife's death than the year before.[4] Other negative states including fear, overwork, anxiety, and physical and mental exhaustion, all summed up by the catch-word 'stress', have the same effect. For example dental and medical students, at times of high stress such as exams, did not make as much protective protein, nor the defensive white cells, although their immunity improved if they practised relaxation every day.[5] Stress, studied both in people and laboratory animals, allows cancers to grow and become more malignant.[6,7]

Other diseases, particularly infections, occur more frequently in people who are stressed and run down.[8,9]

Stress is clearly one culprit for the vulnerability of hospital patients.[10] Another reason, incredibly, is poor food. Malnourishment is one of the signs that a patient will take longer to recover from surgery and is likely to have infections.[11] A recent study of patients who caught infections in hospital found that they were less well nourished, and consumed less vitamins compared with those who did not catch an infection.[12] Despite the considerable body of knowledge that exists on how food and vitamins support health and recovery hospital diets are impoverished. They are especially low in certain vitamins, such as C, and minerals such as zinc.[13]

It turns out that vitamin C and zinc are two food factors which are as lifeblood to the immunity. The white blood cells need a great deal of vitamin C, which they carry around with them to the sites of infection.[14] It is used up in the fight. When there is a lack of vitamin C the immune system is compromised,[15] and vice versa. It has been demonstrated time and again that taking extra vitamin C increases resistance.[16] As for zinc, if it is reduced in the diet the immune organs begin to dry up.[17] Even a marginal lack of zinc has a noticeable effect,[18] and zinc supplements can patch up 'holes' in the resistance due to age or constitution.[19]

Malnutrition, especially of proteins, gives the immune system major stumbling blocks.[11] The white cells are less able to kill invading bacteria, which have a greater chance of gaining ground in the body.[20] People with protein and calorie malnutrition, of the degree commonly met in institutions, have less active white blood cells, and they are more susceptible to viruses, bacteria and fungi.[21] B vitamins and vitamin A are also required by the immune system, especially during disease and stress. They build the barriers to infection in the body tissues, and in the lining of the body's tubes and passages.[22]

Which drugs affect the immune system? Sadly no one really knows because it is hard to check such a thing. Possible lingering side effects such as chronic irritations, a feeling of being run-down, or a shorter life-span, are not investigated. However white blood cells are known to be reduced as a result of antifungal antibiotics such as erythromycin; tricyclic antidepressants; at least one of the nonsteroid anti-inflammatory drugs, namely indomethacin; any preparation containing corticosteroids; and phenothiazine tranquillizers (one in 200 patients severely affected). Any chemotherapeutic agent will have drastic effects on immunity.

Preventing Hospital Infections

To a large extent you are at the mercy of the system once you are in hospital. You cannot become a paranoid, crotchety and anxious patient, worried about a lethal bug behind every curtain, and your immunity suffers from anxiety anyway. But there are a few simple ideas that would seem reasonable:

● Fresh circulating air is important. Try to have as much as possible.
● Don't travel around too much. You don't know what you'll be picking up in the nooks and crannies, and bringing back to bed with you.
● Try to minimize physical contact with other patients.
● Take showers rather than baths.
● Have as much exercise as you can. This is discussed in Chapter 4. Exercise helps lymph vessels to pump their protective fluid round the body. The best exercise for immunity is contracting and relaxing, which you can do as part of a regular progressive relaxation process. Contract and fully relax each part of your body in turn starting from the feet and working upwards. Stretching and deep-breathing exercises are good for the circulation including the lymph.
● If you get a fever in hospital it may be an infection or it may not. Doctors often assume it to be and immediately give antibiotics by drip. However a fever represents the clash of battle and the arousal of your immunity. It sometimes occurs after surgery as part of the clean-up process. Even if it is an infection it may be minor and preferable for you to get over it yourself. Antibiotics, especially the broad-spectrum type, leave you vulnerable for a further infection, perhaps of a more dangerous type.

Therefore if a fever occurs ask that it should not be suppressed by aspirin. Then ask the doctor to check with a microbiologist (an expert on infectious organisms) before giving you antibiotics. Tell him that if it is minor you wish to get over it yourself.

Natural Methods of Bolstering Immunity

There are several ways of helping your immunity to recover from the knocks it receives in hospital, and we will discuss these here. Herbal methods follow in the next section.

Mental Support
Whatever makes you feel well will usually also aid your immunity. This is the raw material for a whole category of folk wisdom. Just as stress reduces immunity, relaxation increases it. This is not an easy

thing to prove, because science is used to looking at the abnormal. Until recently it has only been able to prove that if you are in a poor mental condition your immunity drops. However new studies at the University of Arkansas have demonstrated that the immune reaction to foreign bacteria, measured by a skin test, can be altered by suggestion.[23] Not only that, meditation itself could increase the skin reaction to viruses and the activity of white cells in the blood.[24]

It is not feasible to direct meditation or relaxation towards a goal of improved immunity. You can't feel it. However you can feel the sense of optimism, wellbeing and calm and it is this feeling which is linked to immunity. Therefore use one or other of the methods described in Chapter 4: deep relaxation, autogenics, or yoga breathing and concentration.

Hypnosis and suggestion can be effective in improving the function of the immune system, but only in suggestible patients. In one case people were asked under hypnosis to imagine that their white blood cells were like 'strong powerful sharks with teeth attacking weak confused germ cells in their body'. There resulted a clear increase in white blood cell capability one hour and even one week after the hypnotic suggestion.[25]

Acupuncture and Homeopathy
Both acupuncture and homeopathy can improve immunity. When the gaps in the defences are the result of long-term stress or exhaustion acupuncture can restore the hormones which manage the immunity.[26] We have discussed bringing an acupuncturist or homeopath into hospital to aid recovery, and this aid will include immune support. However the dietary and herbal approach is more directly effective at restoring immunity and preventing infections.

Diet for Defence
The immune system needs to be well stacked up with protein to work best. When it is in the throes of coping with an infection it does not need nutritional help and fasting is one of the best ways of helping the fight. But use protein to build up the defence beforehand. Your meals should contain protein, carbohydrate and fats or oils. But if you can only eat small amounts choose protein rather than carbohydrates: the fish rather than the potatoes.[13]

For carbohydrates make sure you have wholewheat bread, vegetables, or whole grains (e.g. brown rice, not white). These not only give you extra vitamins but help keep your digestion normal when you are lying in bed receiving drugs and treatments that may slow it down. A good digestion and the right intestinal bacteria will help to resist wound infection after surgery.[27]

Eat fresh salads and fresh fruit, which should be organically grown to get the full complement of vitamins and minerals. You need them much more in the hospital than in any other place, and it is advisable to get them brought in, ready-juiced if necessary. Commercial fruit juices are not a substitute as many of the vitamins are long gone and they are loaded with bacteria.[28]

Do not eat a lot of carbohydrate such as bread, potatoes and especially sugar or sweets. Extra carbohydrate is a stress on the system: you need a hormone outburst to digest it, it makes you tired and it is known to depress immunity. It also generates altered blood sugar levels that compromise all parts of the immune system.[29] Remember that you need less lying in bed than doing a day's work, so eat lightly.

Saturated fats inhibit immunity to some extent, partly because they take the place of unsaturated fat, that is fresh oils. There is a good deal of evidence that the performance of certain groups of white blood cells is sensitive to the type of fats in the diet and in the blood.[30] Saturated fats or excess fats of any kind inhibit the cells.[31] Therefore take oils rather than fat or margarine, and if you can get cold-pressed oils so much the better – they contain more of the essential fatty acids that might well be missing from a hospital diet. Above all avoid foods deep fried in old oil or fat – no chips!

Medicinal Foods that Prevent Infections

The queen of preventive remedies is that natural antibiotic, garlic. It is the strongest and best anti-infective agent known outside the pharmacy. You can eat it continuously without fear of harm, and you can be confident it will keep the vampires away as well as the germs. Garlic contains sulphur compounds which are not dissimilar to those of some antibiotics, but it acts as a blunderbuss rather than a rifle, generally preventing the growth of all unusual germs in the body. It has been found effective against very diverse germs including those resistant to modern antibiotics, and nearly a hundred studies going back to Louis Pasteur himself testify to its effect in preventing and curing infections.[32]

It is best to eat garlic fresh although cooked garlic, provided it is crushed, retains a good deal of its medicinal properties. A good preventive dose is one clove three times a day. It can be made more palatable by eating it with salad (especially parsley) or fruit. You may be understandably concerned about the aroma, not wishing to keep the medical staff away along with the vampires. I would venture that the smell is a necessary and very marginal side effect of your own medicine. It might even bring some light relief into the tedious, pervasive smells of Lysol and plastics. However you can get capsules of garlic too. These should not be deodorized garlic which is not of proven effectiveness. Garlic does thin the blood, so it is not advisable to take it before surgery or where there is risk of haemorrhage.

Lactobacillus, taken in tablets or in natural live yoghurt, is a useful protective against intestinal and abdominal infections. It also produces acids in the intestine which stimulate intestinal movement so as to get rid of wastes, and keep the balance of beneficial and vitamin-producing organisms in the intestine.[33] The colon has been described as an immune system all on its own, in so far as it removes poisons and unwanted organisms while retaining the beneficial foods and inhabitants. Lactobacillus helps it work.

Cider vinegar and honey are age-old preventive remedies. They both help to prevent infection in the mouth, throat and digestive tract. Cider vinegar is a good douche or rinse against infections anywhere in the body.

GLA, Gamma Linoleic Acid, is a specific essential fatty acid that acts as a building block for certain local hormones called prostaglandins. These hormones regulate immunity 'in the field', like lieutenants. Supplemental GLA, which can be bought in the form of evening primrose oil or blackcurrant seed oil, can support immunity and general wellbeing, especially if the diet contains saturated, old and questionable fats or oils.[34]

Vitamins and Your Immune System

Defence always seems to take preference in the national budget. Similarly the immune system is demanding of essential nutrients. A lack of virtually all the vitamins (B6, pantothenate, B2, folic acid B2, C, A, and E) and minerals (iron, zinc, calcium, magnesium, iodine and selenium) have been linked with reduced antibody and white cell function.[35]

The better the diet, the fewer vitamin supplements are needed. But as a patient you are not in control of your diet. Cold storage of fruits and vegetables, and cooking all destroy vitamins. Therefore you should insure yourself by supplementation. The most important vitamin supplements are vitamin C, vitamin A, vitamin E, and B complex. For example when unfit adults are given vitamin E (400 IU) and vitamin C (500 mg) daily for some time, the immunological power of their white blood cells increases to match that of fit people.[36]

The best dosage schedule is that suggested in Chapter 4 (page 68). You can substitute yeast for each dose of B vitamins. You should add a daily dose of around 15,000 IU vitamin A if you are not eating fresh carrots or yellow fruit such as peaches and apricots. You must add 15 mg zinc per day unless you are eating a full meal of fish, meat or *free range* eggs, or seeds such as sesame or sunflower seeds.

In the US you can buy supplements specifically to support the immunity. However they are expensive and a hotch-potch; different brands contain radically different mixtures. One, for example, contains vitamin C, zinc, ornithine, selenium, B-carotene and extracts of sheep thymus gland. The advantages of such preparations over the supplementation regime just described are minimal or non-existent, especially if you eat garlic too which ensures extra selenium.

Herbs and Immunity

The real power to aid your immunity exists in the plant kingdom. There is a range of plants under active investigation which can protect and restore your immunity.

Propolis is an anti-infective material which bees collect from the sap of certain trees. They plaster it over the hive where it helps to cleanse the hive and protect young bees from disease. It is a well known folk medicine of Continental and Eastern Europe. Recently Professor Scheller and a team of doctors at the Institute of Microbiology in Zbrze-Kokitinca, Poland, have explored the full range of propolis's effects. Plant-derived substances in propolis called flavonoids are capable of directly stimulating the immune system to make antibodies.[37] They also help white cells to break up potentially harmful bacteria and appear to rejuvenate an immune system that is worn and tired with age or stress. Propolis is harmless. It can be taken every day as a nugget held in the mouth by the gum until eventually dissolved. It is available as tablets.

Mistletoe, *Viscum album*, is a classic plant medicine of Northern Europe, made famous as the holy Druid plant, growing like a transplant on the oak. It is used to lower blood pressure and is a traditional anticancer remedy.[38] However it was noticed that its use in cancer promoted rather than incapacitated immunity.[39] There are sugar-proteins called lectins, plant cell binding materials, which strongly stimulate the cell multiplication of the white blood cells. A team of scientists at the Department of Immunology of the University of Utrecht found that it increases the weight of the organs associated with immunity, the thymus and spleen, and rapidly accelerates the production of antibodies.[40] Mistletoe can be given as a shot in the arm to the immunity, although it should be under the advice of a herbalist. The usual daily dose is 3 gm of powered leaves or 0.5 ml of a tincture.

Herbs used in Western herbalism to promote immunity come under the category of 'alteratives' or 'blood purifiers', lumping together the attacking of an infection with the removal of its products. Three major immune stimulating plants for internal housekeeping are: echinacea (*Echinacea angustifolium*); golden seal

(*Hydrastis canadensis*) and poke (*Phytolacca spp*). These should be taken as powders in capsules, 1 gm three times a day. However for best results the quantity and the plant that is best for you should be determined by prior visit to a herbalist.

The Dramatic Potential of Chinese Herbs

While the West has 100 years of developing drugs that cure diseases, China has several thousand years experience of developing drugs that *prevent* them. While the West values its most powerful agents such as cortisone, the East values mild, safe remedies such as liquorice, calling them kingly remedies. They describe their own strong curative drugs such as ephedra merely as the servants. Chinese medicine is a mirror image of Western medicine because it is based on keeping you healthy and only secondarily curing your ills. In practice this means that many medicines are designed to restore 'holes' in your resistance before they become infections or cancer, to adjust organs before they get out of hand and turn into diabetes or heart disease, to nip stress in the bud before it becomes high blood pressure or migraine, and to adjust the inflammatory temperature of the body before it becomes arthritis.[41]

This prevention and 'tuning' of the body is more difficult than curative medicine. It involves detecting where each person is vulnerable and finding the remedies (or acupuncture points) that work in that subtle manner. But the unbroken development of Chinese culture has allowed an unparalleled sophistication in their medicine. They now know hundreds of plants, each of which can activate, depress, divert, concentrate, disperse or alter any one of a large number of different physiological processes in the body. The immunity, being one of the most critical to health, is of particular interest to Chinese practitioners, and they have discovered many plants that affect it in different ways. We discussed the plants that restore immunity destroyed by chemotherapy and radiotherapy in Chapter 7. Here are some Chinese 'tonic' plants that can be used to strengthen and bolster immunity while you are at risk from less drastic medical circumstances such as a stay in hospital after surgery.

Eleutherococcus senticosus, so-called Siberian ginseng, is a cheaper, less stimulating substitute for *Panax ginseng*, true ginseng. The Russians have developed this plant into one of their major medicines, entered it into their pharmacopoeia, and distribute 12 million bottles a month. Some of this is used in hospitals to 'normalize' blood pressure and metabolism after the shock of treatment. They describe its action as adaptogenic, that is helping the body to regulate itself, and to deal with stress. I have over a hundred Soviet studies on *Eleutherococcus* from research institutes and hospitals.[42]

The immune-protective and immune-stimulating properties of *Eleutherococcus* had long been suspected by Soviet scientists, based on their laboratory tests. This led to an enormous trial in which it was given to 60,000 workers at the Volzhsky car factory in Togliatti.[43] There was a dramatic reduction in the usual infections. Researchers at the Institute of Materia Medica of the Chinese Academy of Sciences have isolated a substance from *Eleutherococcus* which can activate white blood cells and generally strengthen immunity, and they are preparing to produce this material as a medicine.[44]

Angelica sinensis (Dang Kwei) is described as the 'female ginseng' in that it is recommended for restoring energy and vitality, but in females rather than males, for whom regular ginseng is better. It has been found to have strong immune protective effects, by activating different kinds of white cells and antibody-forming spleen cells.[45] It is one of the best specific stimulants of a threatened immunity, but is not strong enough for use after chemotherapy.

Liquorice can be very effective, surprisingly, at promoting antibody production and the regulation of white cells. However it can also, under certain conditions, depress the immunity, so it should only be taken for immune defence in a professionally prepared herb mixture. It is an excellent general tonic after illness.[46]

Panax ginseng, true ginseng, is the best recovery medicine there is, particularly in cases of severe debility, loss of energy, poor hormone function, poor immune function, and weakness from disease. It increases the number of white cells in the blood, increases their general responsiveness, and helps spleen and liver provide energy for immunological reactions. It is described more fully in Chapter 4. Ginseng is rather stimulating if it is good quality, and worthless if it is not.[47] The stimulation is valuable when you are weak and getting back on your feet, for example after surgery. There are also situations where you do not need stimulation, for example healthy people with psychiatric problems, or people in hospital for some organic conditions. *Panax ginseng* is also contraindicated in the case of inflammations and acute illnesses.

A plant that is used as a substitute for ginseng and is of considerable benefit to the immunity is *Codonopsitis lanceolate,* or Tang-Shen. It is not stimulating but nourishes the immunity.

Note: American ginseng (*Panax quinquefolium*) can be used at any time as a non-stimulating and even slightly sedative general tonic. Its effects on immunity have not been investigated, but judging from traditional sources and the nature of the plant constituents I suspect it has a good deal of the immune-restoring qualities of *Panax ginseng.*[47]

Availability

You will be able to find *Panax ginseng* and American ginseng,

Eleutherococcus, liquorice and perhaps Dang Kwei in your local health shop. Take 1 gm two or three times a day. I have purposely left out many immune stimulating and restorative Chinese herbs which are not yet available in the West. However you can get certain mixtures commercially and they combine different complementary Chinese tonic herbs so that the total is much better than the sum of its parts. For example ginseng may provide energy, but when combined with ginger it aids the circulation so that the effects of ginseng are spread properly, while added liquorice regulates water balance, to harmonize the other two. Chinese companies export some mixtures, such as Shou Wu Chih (a source of angelica) or Peking Royal Jelly Liquid (a source of codonopsitis together with Royal Jelly, a useful tonic in its own right) or Shih Chuan Ta Pu Tonic Pills (a mixture of the best Oriental herbs for immune support). There are some American-made products beginning to appear. Generally, of the products which mention immune support, choose those consisting of Chinese herbal mixtures as they will be most effective.

REFERENCES

1. Internal Medical News, reported in People's Medical Society newsletter of February 1985.
2. *The Observer* 31 August 1986 quoting Dr. Jean Bradley.
3. Simanowitz, A. *J. Hospital Infection,* **5** (Supplement A) 117–119 (1984).
4. Schleifer, S. J. *et al, J. American Medical Assoc.,* **250** 374–377 (1983).
5. Kiecolt-Glaser, J. N. *et al, Psychosomatic Medicine,* **46** 7–14 (1984); Wood, C. *New Scientist,* 31, (4 July 1985).
6. Fox, B. H. and Newberry, B. H. (eds.), *Impact of Psychoendocrine Systems in Cancer and Immunity,* C. S. Hogrefe, Lewiston N.J. (1984).
7. Greer H. S. and Morris, T. *J. Psychosomatic Res.* **19** 147–153 (1975).
8. Editorial, *The Lancet,* **2** 133 (1985).
9. Bieliauskar, L. A. *Stress and its Relationship to Health and Illness,* Westview Press, Boulder, Colorado (1982).
10. Boore, J. R. P. *Prescription for Recovery,* Royal College of Nursing, London (1978).
11. Garibaldi, R. A. *et al, Am. J. Medicine,* **70** 677–680 (1981).
12. Unpublished Paper, *Division of Hospital Infection,* Central Public Health Laboratory, London NW9 5HT.
13. Chandra, R. K. *Nutrition Reviews,* **39** 225–231 (1981); Levy, J. A. In: Stites *et al,* (eds.) *Basic and Clinical Immunity,* 297–305, Los Altos, CA. Lange Medical, (1982).
14. Stamkova, L. *et al, Infection and Immunity,* **12** 252–6 (1975); Drutz, D. J. and Mills, J. In: Stites, *et al,* (eds.) *Basic and Clinical Immunity,* 209–232, Los Altos, CA. Lange Medical, (1982).

15. Ismail, A. H. *et al, Federation Proceedings,* **42** (3) Abstract 252 (1983). Fraser, R. C. *et al, Am. J. Clinical Nutr.,* **33** 839–847 (1978).
16. Basu, T. K. and Schorah, C. J. *Vitamin C in Health and Disease,* Croom Helm, London (1981); Prinz, W. *et al, Int. J. Vit. Nutr. Res.,* **47** 248–257 (1977).
17. Gallin, J. I. and Fauci, A. S. (eds.) *Advances in Host Defense Mechanisms,* 275–359, Plenum Press, N.Y. (1983); Tanaka, T. *et al,* Fed. Proceedings, **37** 931 (1978); Fernandes, G. *et al,* Proc. Nat. Acad. Sci., **87** 725–8 (1977).
18. Fabris, N. *et al, Lancet,* **1** 983–6 (1984).
19. Duchateau, *et al, Am. J. Clinical Nutr.,* **34** 88–93 (1981); Wagner, P. A. *et al, Int. J. Vit. Nutr. Res.,* **53** 94–101 (1983).
20. Sobrado, J. *et al, Am. J. Clinical Nutr.,* **37** 795–801 (1983).
21. Chandra, R. K. *The Lancet,* **I** 688–691 (1983).
22. Chandra, R. K. *World Rev. Nutrition Dietetics,* **25** 166–188 (1976).
23. Smith, R. G. *Psychosomatic Med.,* **46** 65–70 (1983).
24. Smith, R. G. *et al, Arch. Int. Med.,* **145** 2110–2112 (1985); Hildenbrand, G. *J. Alt. Med.,* 16–23 (February 1986).
25. Hall, H. R. *Am. J. Clinical Hypnosis,* **25** 92–101 (1983).
26. Ding, V. *et al, Am. J. Acup.,* 51–4 (1983); Steidler, N. E., **11** *Abstracts,* No. 173 (1983).
27. Loniseau, quoted in ref. 10.
28. Schimpff, S. C. *Infectious Diseases,* **144** 81–84 (1981).
29. Anderson, K. E. *et al, Nutrition Rev.,* **40** 161–171 (1982).
30. Wardle, E. N. *Lancet,* **2** 423 (1976); Nordenstrom, J. *et al, Am. J. Clinical Nutr.,* **32** 2416–2422 (1979).
31. Hawley, H. P. and Gordon. G. B. *Laboratory Investigation,* **34** 216–222 (1976); Chandra, R. K. *Am. J. Clin. Nutrition,* **33** 13–16 (1980); Berken, A. and Benacerraf, B. *Proc. Soc. Exp. Biol. Med.,* **128** 793–5 (1968).
32. For a full survey of the medical evidence see: Blackwood, J. and Fulder, S. *Garlic: Nature's Original Remedy,* Javelin Books, Poole, Dorset (1986).
33. Rasic, J. L. and Kurmann, J. A. *Bifidobacteria and their Role,* Birkhauser Verlag (1983).
34. Horrobin, D. F. (ed.), *Clinical Uses of Essential Fatty Acids,* Eden Press, London (1982).
35. For summaries of the evidence see: Dickenson, D. *How to Fortify Your Immune System,* Arlington Books, London (1982).
36. Ismail, A. H. *et al, Fed. Proc.,* **42** Abstract, 252 (1983).
37. Wade, C. *Let's Live,* 26 (March 1985).
38. Anderson, L. A. *Pharmaceutical Journal,* 437–439 (16 October 1982).
39. Nienhaus, J. *et al, Experientia,* **26** 523 (1970).
40. Bloksma, N. *et al, Planta Medica,* **46** 221–227 (1982).
41. See Fulder, S. *The Tao of Medicine: Ginseng, Oriental Remedies and the Pharmacology of Harmony,* Destiny, N.Y. (1982).
42. Brekhman, I. I. *Man and Biologically Active Substances,* Pergamon Press, Oxford and N.Y. (1980).
43. Galanova, G. K. In: Brekhman, I. I. (ed), *Adaptation and Adaptogens,* 126–127, Vladivostok, USSR Academy of Sciences (1977).

44. Peigen, X. *J. of Ethnopharmacology,* **7** 95–109 (1983).
45. Shanghai Inst. of Materia Medica *Kexue Tobao,* **24** 764, (1979).
46. Kumagai, A. and Takata, M. *Proc. Symp. Wakan Yaku,* **11** 79–83 (1978).
47. Fulder, S. *About Ginseng,* Thorsons, U.K. (1976).

CHAPTER 9

Drugs and their Side Effects

During the last century the herbalists, or Galenicists as they were then called, mounted a vigorous attack on the chemists or chymists. They accused them of selling harmful remedies which were discovered in the laboratory, by accident, and which teated only the symptoms, leaving the disease itself to fester. Their lack of therapeutic principles led Voltaire to accuse physicians of prescribing 'medicines of which they know little, to cure diseases of which they know less in human beings of which they know nothing.'

But the chymists won hands down. They took some of the herbalists' materials and a little of their knowledge into the laboratory, and out came chemicals which did spectacular things to symptoms. Aspirin, from witch hazel, made fevers plummet, digoxin, from foxglove, kept hearts pumping regularly. The public rushed to welcome the new miracle remedies, and the herbalists warnings were, for the moment, forgotten.

Today, after thalidomide and steroids, after a generation which has been taking more and more drugs and not getting healthier as a result, even your average high street medical practitioner may concede that the Galenicists had a point. Drugs are discovered by virtue of noticeable effects they have on animals. Therefore only the strong ones, which clearly make a rat's whiskers twitch, are selected. They are sold before they have built a tradition of safe use in human society (most safety testing is done in laboratory mice society).

Take for example codeine, a common constituent of the plethora of cough medicines on the market. It stops coughing, indeed, but as it is developed for use against the symptom, not to heal the person, the real results are unwanted effects. It keeps the mucous in the lungs making recovery slower than it would be otherwise. It causes constipation and tiredness, and puts stress on the liver.

UK doctors have 4,000 drugs to choose from, which consume 10% of the national medical bill, at great profit to the manufacturers. One in two adults take a drug every day in the industrialized nations.[1] During illness almost every child takes at least one drug every day, and if you are in hospital the chances are you will be given one more drug every other day.[2] Three quarters of all visits to a GP will end with a prescription.[3]

With all this consumption, and with the drugs being such blunt instruments, it is inevitable that major catastrophies have occurred through drug side effects. A leading paper in the *Journal of the American Medical Asociation* in 1950 was entitled 'Little Evidence that Huge Amounts of DES (Diethylstilbestrol) Harm Pregnant Women or Their Babies'. Nearly 35 years later another paper in the same journal was entitled 'Increased Incidence of Cervical and Vaginal Dysplasia (i.e. cancer) in 3980 DES Exposed Young Women'.[4] Sulphonamides, the precursors of modern antibiotics, were widely used to protect normal premature babies in hospital from infections, until it was realized that they caused brain damage. Thalidomide was an apparently harmless sedative. Millions of people took the apparently harmless bacteria-killing drug clioquinol, (enterovioform) for 'holiday tum' until thousands of Japanese became permanently and painfully disabled after the drug ate away their nerves.

The drastic side effects caused by such drugs would be more understandable if the drugs were a vital contribution to health, i.e., if we know there is no alternative and the risks have been explained. No one is going to sue a drug company for loss of hair during chemotherapy. But much of the side effect problem is the result of drugs which are more or less unnecessary. In the above examples coughs, a good night's sleep, holiday tummy and to some extent the vulnerability of premature babies (see Chapter 13) are all treatable by natural methods of self-care.

In fact only 10% of the drugs now consumed in the industrial nations are for real diseases. People 'swallow hundreds of tons of pharmaceutical products, presumably for relief from the almost incurable disease of being alive'.[5] In some cases this habit is lethal.

Here are a few alarming statistics relating to drug use:

● The massive Boston Collaborative Drug Survey has monitored 19,000 hospital patients and found that one third suffer from adverse effects of drugs.[6]
● The most common drug side effects are from tranquillizers, sedatives, antibiotics, diuretics, painkillers, heart drugs, steroids and anti-inflammatory drugs.
● One in 200 hospital patients die from drug effects.[2] More people die from adverse effects in the US than are killed on the roads.[7]
● Costs of dealing with drug side effects is put at $3 billion in the US.[8]
● In the UK 33% of men and 40% of women have to use drugs

constantly (contraceptives apart) for a chronic health problem.
● About seven prescriptions are filled per person per year in the West.

Background on Side Effects

When you take a drug, for example for high blood pressure, it is designed to have a specific effect on a certain body process, in this case blocking the arousing or 'pump-hard' messages that arrive at the heart. But everything in the body is interconnected. Thus messages to the heart also open the airways to the lungs, and drugs that block these messages may therefore cause asthma as a side effect. Though scientists try and make the drugs as specific as possible, for example by trying to design the drug key to fit the heart lock and not the lungs lock, they are only partially successful. The drugs have a powerful effect on the heart and a lesser effect everywhere else.

At the same time, drugs are continually eliminated from the body through the kidneys' producing urine, and through the liver by chemical breakdown. The healthier these waste-disposal systems, the less damage is done to the body by drugs. The lower the dosage, the less unintended effects the drugs will have, and the more chance there is for the disposal systems to clear them out.

All drugs are poisons to a greater or lesser extent. There is no such thing as a completely harmless drug. But whether or not you will get a noticeable side effect depends on dosage, kidney and liver function, constitution, general health and resistance, age, diet, and many other factors. Doctors can never predict who will get which side effect. It is also a question of sensitivity. A healthy person may feel a side effect which is not felt by his unhealthy cousin. It may be that he is more aware of what's going on inside. Even if drug side effects are not noticeable as a symptom, it doesn't mean that they are not there. They may only appear later, as with antibiotics and vulnerability to subsequent infections. Or they may appear when the dose is raised or when an additional drug is taken. For example tinnitus, ringing in the ear, is a very common and mild side effect. In the US 36 million people have it, often from barbiturates and diuretics. It tends to turn up when tobacco, alcohol or coffee are taken as well as the medical drug. Susceptible people tend to have smaller blood vessels bringing blood and nutrients to the inner ear.

Your doctor should be on the lookout for bad reactions to drugs. Unfortunately it is not always easy to distinguish drug reactions from symptoms of the disease or a new disease, especially when those reactions are unusual. Doctors often believe the assurances of nice-sounding package literature supplied by the pharmaceutical industry and can't believe what they see. For example patients who had severe side effects to their eyes and intestinal organs from the blood pressure lowering drug practolol were for years being given more drugs against supposed neuroses, anxiety, migraines, multiple sclerosis, etc., until the truth eventually dawned on their doctors. Doctors are often lulled into a false sense of security concerning the drugs that have been in common use for some time. But they should not be. Clioquinol had been used for 40 years before cases of nerve degeneration and paralysis began to be reported in the medical literature. Even then it took 8 years before the drug was stopped.

Side effects, especially of new drugs, are meant to be reported to the authorities, but not more than 1% of side effects are reported by doctors. It is scandalous that patients are not trusted enough to be permitted to report side effects directly to the medicines authorities (the Committee of Safety of Medicines of the DHSS) in the UK. Neither are there laymen, i.e. consumers' representatives, on this committee.

If you report an unacceptable side effect to your doctor he will often replace the drug with a similar one, or change the dosage schedule. Sometimes you can be given further drugs to cope with the side effects, as antihistamines, sedatives or tranquillizers are given to people with tinnitus. There are, however, very few actual drug antidotes to other drugs; the doctor's strategy will always be to try and deal with whatever symptoms turn up one by one, with the general health of the patient often becoming worse and worse as each new drug is added. Surprisingly, conventional medicine knows almost nothing about dietary methods of hastening the removal and detoxification of drugs.

How To Avoid Drug Side Effects

The best guards against drug side effects are good prescribing habits in the doctor, watchfulness and awareness in the patient, and a tacit agreement between the two that drugs should not be a first resort.

Your doctor should not be conditioned to reach for the prescription pad when he sees you. He should have a healthy respect for all drugs, and express a wish to cut prescribing to the barest essentials. We discussed your doctor in Chapter 2.

You must tell your doctor you don't like to take drugs. He may assume the opposite unless you make it very clear.

Your doctor should not prescribe an unfamiliar new drug if there is an older well-established one available. If you hear 'I want to try a new medicine that looks very promising' ask what's wrong with the old one.

The doctor should know, and tell you, why this drug is chosen, what benefit he expects from it, what to do if there is no benefit, what problems may occur and how to deal with them. Much unnecessary drugging results from doctors not having a *clear aim* in mind when prescribing and not having the ability to assess if the target has been reached.

You should discuss with the doctor whether the remedy actually cures the disease or whether it only relieves the symptoms, and if so for how long. Ask what will happen then, and whether you will then have to raise the dosage.

Ask yourself and your doctor whether the drug really is necessary. Will the problem go away by itself anyway? Is it trivial? Ask yourself if you are going to the doctor more as a conditioned reflex and whether a drug is not actually the answer you need. If you feel the weight of modern life, will a tranquillizer really lift it, or will it make you more helpless? Is it better to eat more salads and greens for life or be on laxatives for life? Are the blood pressure drugs worth it or is it better to try and change a few habits?

Try preventive methods of treating common non-serious ailments before exploring the drug option. Many frequent symptoms such as tension-headache, sore throat, frequent colds and infections, digestive upsets, skin irritations, anxiety, mild depression or circulatory problems in their early stages are very successfully treated by a change in diet, more exercise and fresh air, reducing the pollution inside your body, psychological work, relaxation and massage. Complementary medicine is another option, to create in you the conditions for health so that you will have no need of any drugs.

Discuss your life style with the doctor. Will the drugs interfere with driving, your intellectual or physical work, your job? If so can they be taken in a different way, or can different drugs, or a drugless solution to the problem be substituted?

Your Ten Questions
1. What is the drug called? What type of drug is it? (the first gives you the brand name e.g. Tetrex, the second question should give you the generic name, e.g. tetracycline).
2. What does the drug do?
3. Why do I need it?
4. What will happen if I don't take it?
5. Will I be able to stop taking it easily?
6. When and how should I take it?
7. What are the possible side effects? What might happen?
8. How long should I take it for and when should I see results?
9. Are there any foods, drinks, supplements or over-the-counter

medicines I shouldn't take or that I should take?
10 When do you want to see me again?

When You Buy and Take Drugs

● Never assume that a drug is harmless and it won't hurt to try it.
A completely harmless drug is yet to be invented.
● Never assume that if a little works then more will work better.
● A mixture of ingredients is not necessarily better than a single
one and may be more toxic.
● When you buy a drug over-the-counter (OTC) at the
pharmacy/drug store make sure you know the answers to questions
1, 2, 5–9. If not, ask the pharmacist.
● Keep to the doctor's or pharmacist's instructions on how to take
your drug. If he says take it with meals three times a day, do just
that: it will minimize harmful effects.
● If you are in doubt take a drug with food rather than without.
● Don't use old drugs. They may have lost their value and some,
such as tetracyclines, can be more harmful when old.

Watching for Drug Side Effects

You need to be on the lookout for unwanted effects. You cannot leave
that to your doctor. Be aware of any changes in symptoms, or
feelings, even subtle ones like irritability, dryness in your mouth,
itching, or tiredness. They may be signs that something is not going
well – the tip of the iceberg of invisible damage being created in your
body.

A very useful tool for watching what's going on is a diary. Make a
daily note of how you feel and whether your original problem is
disappearing or new ones are appearing. Sometimes the months pass,
and you may just get used to being ill, without realizing that you are
now suffering from drug effects different from your original problem.

Here is a check list of symptoms that are frequently produced by
drugs. It may help you to focus accurately on anything that crops up.

Do You Have Any of These Symptoms While Taking Drugs?

Affected Part	Symptom	Affected Part	Symptom
Eyes	Double vision	Muscles	Muscle pain esp. neck
	Watering		Muscle cramps
	Blurred vision		Muscle weakness
	Yellowing of whites		Tremors or shakes
			Numbness

Do You Have Any of These Symptoms While Taking Drugs?

Affected Part	Symptom	Affected Part	Symptom
Ears and Nose	Ringing in ears	Digestion	Dry mouth
	Pain in ears		Loss of appetite
	Bad smells/tastes		Diarrhoea
Skin	Itch		Unusual thirst
	Rash		Nausea or vomiting
	Flushing		Stomach pain
	Yellowing		Bloody or black stools
	Unusual sweating	Urine	Incontinence
	Feeling of insects crawling		Painful or frequent urination
Mind and Head	Irritability		Cloudy or dark urine
	Dizziness		
	Fainting	General	Unexpected fevers
	Frequent yawning		Chills
	Apathy and lethargy		Puffiness, esp. hands, feet
	Unsteadiness		Swelling
	Headaches		Unexpected weight loss or gain
	Depression		
	Lack of concentration		Unusual menstruation or heavy bleeding
	Insomnia		
	Loss of memory		Loss of sexual drive
	Panic		Impotence
	Hallucinations		
	Hyperactivity		
Chest and Throat	Constricted throat		
	Breathlessness		
	Unusually rapid or slow heartbeat		
	Chest pain		
	Palpitations		

Obtaining Further Information

Your doctor may not tell you what you want to know; perhaps he doesn't know himself. It may be that the doctor doesn't believe that you have side effects, or doesn't understand how you feel. It is not always apparent to patients how much a doctor is subtly guided and influenced by drug companies who are always keen to play down their drugs' disadvantages. A survey recently pointed out that 11 out of 28 advertisements in the *British Medical Journal* on 17/11/1984 were in breach of the UK Medicines Law.[11] In other words your doctor too might be duped, even if he has the best intentions.

In such cases you may need independent information on the drug you are taking. The classical sources of information are the Physicians Desk Reference (PDR) in the US and the British National Formulary

(BNF) in the UK. These are available in the libraries, and your doctor will have up-to-date copies. Look up the drug in the index and check the contra-indications (situations in which the drug must not be prescribed), adverse effects and other information. Try to get your doctor or the pharmacist to give you the leaflet or package insert enclosed with the drug. This will be phrased in medical terminology, but with the help of a medical dictionary, or even a good ordinary dictionary, most of the words are translatable. Asking for the package insert need not seem an outrageous question. A US 'Patient Package Insert' programme was given priority during President Carter's administration. Many authorities have been pleading for clear, simple package inserts to be given to every patient. After all, 'It is the co-operative patient not the compliant patient who has the best chance for safe and effective therapy. Of course only adequately informed patients can be expected to be co-operative.'[12]

A Note on Drug Naming

It is important to understand how drugs are named so that when you ask your doctor what those pink ones were you will understand his answer. You will also need this information for the coming chapters.

Drugs are classed broadly into purposes for which they are used. Let us look at drugs against infection:

Some purposes of anti-infective drugs
To kill bacteria
To kill viruses
To kill fungus etc.

There are several types of chemical substances used for each purpose:

Some chemical types of drugs which kill bacteria
The penicillins
The tetracyclines
The aminoglycosides
The sulphonamides etc.

There may be several specific chemicals to choose from within each chemical type. The specific chemical is otherwise known as the *generic* name of the drug:

Some choices within the penicillin type
ampicillin
benzyl penicillin
methicillin
amoxycillin etc.

There may be more than one drug product made by the pharmaceutical companies containing the specific chemical. Each has a *brand* name:

Some brands of ampicillin
Amfipen
Penbritin
Ampilar
Vidopen etc.

To know your drug you need to know its purpose (e.g. killing bacteria, or 'antibacterial'), its chemical type (one of the penicillins) and its brand name (e.g. Penbritin). The British National Formulary can help you to distinguish the names of each drug.

Stopping Medical Drugs

Supposing you are having adverse effects which are unacceptable and you have decided to stop taking a medical drug, what should you do? People often just stop taking drugs without telling their doctors. This is patronizingly called 'non-compliance' by the medical profession – not doing what you are told. Two out of 5 people do not take their medicines as directed, or at all, mostly because of side effects. They are very often the lucky ones! But there are a few things you should know before you throw your drugs out of the window.

Very often the symptoms that made you take the drugs in the first place will come back twice as hard when you stop them. Therefore you should be prepared to put something in their place, either complementary medicine, self-care or a complete break in your usual routine. For example stopping laxatives may bring on greater constipation than before, requiring a thorough dietary change. Stopping decongestants and nasal sprays may make your nasal passages more stuffed up than they were before, and you may need to go to a homeopath or herbalist for relief.

In the case of some prescribed drugs the suppressed symptoms return with such force that you put your life at risk if you stop suddenly. This is the case with drugs for the circulation, psychiatric and mood-altering drugs, muscle-relaxants, anti-epileptic drugs and others. In other cases, particularly steroids, the drugs have made important functions of the body redundant, so the drugs cannot be withdrawn immediately. There are also cases, particularly with antibiotics or anticancer drugs, where withdrawal in mid-course can worsen the disease. Your doctor will be able to advise you on any risks of stopping the drugs. Where there are risks the drugs should be tailed off gradually with the help of a complementary therapist or holistic practitioner who can substitute safer treatment bit by bit.

Where there is no risk the drugs can indeed be thrown away. But do it properly: don't express your reluctance to take drugs by taking them in an erratic on-off manner. You are safer taking drugs properly or not at all.

Which Vitamins Should I Take to Help Prevent Drug Side Effects?

A good deal of knowledge has now been gathered on the interconnections between drugs and dietary factors. Many drugs remove vitamins from the body, by using them up, or by preventing their absorbtion in the digestion from food you eat, or by killing bacteria in the intestine on which you depend. Some of the drug side effects are the result of a lack of vitamins caused by drugs. For example barbiturates put a load on the liver and disturb the machinery there which makes Vitamin D ready for the bones. Bone weakness produced by using barbiturates for long periods can be prevented by Vitamin D.[13] Many drugs gradually weaken the kidney leading to a profound lack of vitality and general health. This deterioration can be partly prevented by a diet rich in potassium, magnesium and Vitamin B_6.[14] Cases of tiredness, loss of memory, confusion and irritation that arise from drugs can sometimes be relieved by B vitamins.

Mineral depletion also occurs with some drugs, either because they affect the kidney, making it a leaky sieve (e.g. diuretics), or because they prevent proper absorbtion from the food (e.g. laxatives), or because the stomach wall is damaged (e.g. neomycin).

The specific vitamin and mineral losses are given in the following tables. Your doctor may not know about all these vitamin losses: he may not have read the relevant literature.[15] You should take above the Daily Recommended Allowance of the vitamins concerned, and spread the dosage throughout the day, roughly in parallel with drug dosage.

In some of these cases (see p. 166) vitamins can protect against the supersensitivity of those who react especially badly to drugs. For example certain people have side effects of asthma and rashes arising from aspirin and other anti-inflammatory drugs used in rheumatic diseases. French scientists gave one group of sensitive people 1 gm of Vitamin C and 600 mg Vitamin E per day before, during and after drug treatment. The side effects were completely abolished compared with other sensitive patients who received look-alike inert pills instead of the vitamins.[16]

DRUGS THAT DEPLETE VITAMINS[15]

Type of Drug	Purpose of Drug	Vitamin depleted
anticonvulsants, esp. phenytoin	prevent epileptic seizures	D, K, Folic Acid, B6
antacids	reduce stomach acidity	A, B complex
aspirin (and salicylates)	reduce pain, fever, inflammation	A, C, E, K
barbiturates	sedatives, sleeping pills	A, D, Folic Acid, C
cholestyramine	lowers cholesterol in blood	A, D, K, Folic Acid, B complex, B12
clofibrate	lowers cholesterol in blood	K
colchicine	treats gout	B12, A
corticosteroids	prevent inflammations and allergies	A, B6, D, C
diuretics	increase urination	B complex
estrogen-type contraceptives	contraception (the 'pill')	Folic Acid, B6, B12, B2
epsom salts	cleanse the bowels	B2, K
hydralazine	lowers blood pressure	B6
indomethacin	used in rheumatism and arthritis	B1, C
isoniazid	treats tuberculosis	B6, B3
levo-dopa	treats Parkinson's disease	B6
mineral oil	laxative	A, D, K
neomycin	treats bacterial infections	B12, A
nitrofurantoin	treats bacterial infections of the urinary systems	Folic Acid
penicillamine	treats rheumatoid arthritis	B6
phenothiazine	treats psychosis and schizophrenia	B2
potassium chloride	used in potassium deficiency	B12
pyrimethamine	prevention and treatment of malaria	Folic Acid
sulphasalazine	treats ulcerative colitis	Folic Acid
tetracycline	kills bacteria	C
trimethoprim + sulphonamides	kills bacteria	Folic Acid, K, B

DRUGS THAT DEPLETE MINERALS[15]

Type of Drug	Purpose of Drug	Mineral depleted
anticonvulsants	prevent epileptic seizures	calcium
antacids	reduce stomach acidity	phosphate
aspirin	reduces pain, fever, inflammation	iron, phosphate

DRUGS THAT DEPLETE MINERALS[15] (contd.)

Type of Drug	Purpose of Drug	Mineral depleted
barbiturates	induce sleeping	phosphates
chemotherapeutic drugs	treat cancerous growth	magnesium, zinc
colchicine	treats gout	sodium, calcium, potassium, iron
cortisone	prevents inflammation	calcium, potassium
diuretics	increase urination	potassium, magnesium, zinc
laxatives	reduce constipation	potassium, calcium
neomycin	kills bacteria	sodium, potassium, calcium, iron

There are also certain rare cases where you should not take vitamins with medication because they counteract it.[15] This is why you should inform your doctor about the vitamins you are taking. Cases include:

Type of Drug	Purpose of Drug	Vitamin
anticoagulants	risk of blood clots	Vit. K or large amounts of leafy vegetables reduce effect
anti-psychotic drugs	psychoses	Vit. C can reduce effect
levodopa	Parkinson's disease	B6 and B complex reduce effect
methotrexate	leukaemia	Folic Acid, B2, can reduce effect
sulphonamides	urinary infections	Vit. C can cause kidney stones
tetracyclines	infections	Iron, milk, reduce absorbtion

Dietary Methods of Combating Drug Side Effects

There is an interplay between foods and drugs at three levels. There are interactions immediately when food is taken with drugs so as to delay or accelerate absorbtion. Food can also affect the quantities of drug in the body, how long it takes to be eliminated and the side effects. Lastly food can help in eliminating after effects and toxic accumulations, and restoring health after you have stopped taking drugs.

Taking Foods with Drugs

Food in the stomach will slow down the absorbtion of most drugs. In consequence the amount of the drug in the body at any one time will be reduced. This may or may not be desirable depending on the drug. If aspirin is taken with food it takes much longer to have an effect, but food will protect the wall of the stomach from attack by aspirin. Some drugs are weaker when taken with food because they become stuck to food components, for example the heart-stimulating drug digoxin on bran, and tetracyclines on milk. Some examples are:

Better Absorbed on Empty Stomach	*Better Absorbed on Full Stomach*
cephalexin (antibiotic)	anticoagulants (prevent blood clotting)
cimetidine (treats stomach ulcer)	
digoxin (stimulates heart beat)	chlorothiazide (increases urination)
erythromycin (antibiotic)	griseofulvin (treats fungal infections)
metronidazole (treats amoebic and other infections)	nitrofurantoin (treats urinary infections)
penicillin (antibiotic)	propanolol (treats fungal infections)
tetracycline (antibiotic)	tranquillizers
theophylline (relieves bronchitis and asthma)	

Milk is a good medium for taking some drugs as it protects the stomach. But do not take tetracycline with milk. Do not take penicillin and other antibiotics with fruit juices as the acid may break up the drug prematurely.

Foods Protecting the Body from Drug Side Effects

Your body should be in a condition where it takes drug chemicals to pieces and gets them out quickly after they have done their job. A hit-and-run action will give your body a chance for drug-free spaces. The key organs which dispose of drugs are the liver and kidney.

The liver has a number of catalysts which break up all incoming foreign chemicals, waste products of the metabolism, body messengers which have given their message and come to the liver to be 'shredded' and so on. These waste-disposal systems are vital to health and are much abused in the modern world by endless and excessive rubbish such as drugs, food additives, pollutants, car exhausts, pesticides, and so on. The waste-disposal systems only have a certain capacity. If this is exceeded poisons spill over and damage the liver itself, something that happens frequently during long-term use of drugs. For example therapeutic doses of the painkiller paracetamol are disposed of very well by liver catalysts. But this process needs an important housekeeping material called glutathione. If too much paracetamol is taken and all the glutathione is used up, the rest of the paracetamol goes on a destructive rampage through the liver destroying tissue. People taking paracetamol overdoses are treated in hospital with cysteine or cysteamine, which create more glutathione.

Drugs which can damage the liver include paracetamol in high doses, sulphonamides (treat infections), salicylates (relieve pain and inflammation), rifampicin (treats tuberculosis), tetracyclines (antibiotics), cancer chemotherapeutic drugs, halothane-type anaesthetics, isoniazid (treats tuberculosis), phenothiazines (treat psychoses and schizophrenia), many steroids including oral contraceptives, drugs against diabetes and drugs against thyroid problems.

You should support the liver while taking any medical drugs, in particular the above. One way is to take foods rich in selenium, vitamin C and vitamin E. These antioxidant food factors will maintain the level of the glutathione waste system in the liver. Vitamin C is present in fresh fruit and vegetables. Garlic, onion and, to a lesser extent, radish and horseradish contain both selenium and compounds not unlike cysteine which will help maintain the glutathione. Garlic has been proved to protect the liver from damage by chemicals.[18]

Catalysts in the liver which dispose of drugs are primed by certain food components, particularly the cabbage family, which includes broccoli, Brussels sprouts, cauliflower and spring greens as well as all kinds of cabbage.[19] Other similarly helpful components (termed flavonoids) are found in lemons.

Specific herbs which aid the liver in its clean-up are discussed below. But many aromatic and resinous spice plants are helpful to the liver and should not be forgotten in the diet. These include fennel, dill, ginger, cinnamon and pepper. A native doctor once treated me for poisoning in Lahore, Pakistan. His remedy was nothing more nor less than a bowlful of very hot mango pickle. I managed to work my way through it, with much sighing and sweating, and indeed the expected symptoms were prevented.

In general terms the liver is protected by a low-fat, alcohol-free, additive-free and nutritious diet.

A healthy kidney is just as important for removal of drugs as the liver, and it is even more sensitive to damage by drugs. Almost every drug can affect the kidney, sometimes irreversibly, as they leave the body. The kidney is supported by B vitamins such as B6, and by the best possible environment in the inner sea bathing the tissues of the body. The body water should be made slightly alkaline by alkaline foods particularly vegetables, salads and grains rather than acids such as sugars and starches. Sufficient magnesium and potassium will help the kidney eliminate drugs. These are found in seeds, nuts and green leafy vegetables and salads, preferably organically grown. You should also drink a lot of water and juices to help the kidney filter out the poisons. Vegetable juices would combine all the above requirements. The kidney is also protected by a low-protein diet.

Quite a few drugs are also eliminated by the bile and through the digestion. To help in the elimination of these drugs you need a diet with plenty of roughage, and a helpful normal bacterial zoo in the intestine. This implies an increase in plant protein at the expense of animal protein, and grains, i.e. as much of a natural wholefood semi-vegetarian diet as possible, with plenty of fruit.

Summarizing the above, here are some nutritional guidelines to help in drug elimination and to protect your kidneys and liver:

● Avoid alcohol, refined oils, animal fats, extra salt, additives, preservatives, chemicals of any kind and smoking.
● Take 1 gm vitamin C, 200 IU vitamin E and 100 mg. vitamin B complex (make sure it has B6 as a major component) twice a day.
● Drink vegetable juices and fruit juices plus pure water totalling at least 1½ litres a day.
● Eat root vegetables, dark green leafy vegetables especially the cabbage family, salads, alfalfa and other sprouts, garlic and onion. But discuss your diet with your doctor if you are taking anticoagulants.
● Eat lentils, grains, seeds (e.g. sunflower, sesame or pumpkin), soya products, beans, fish and liver.
● Supplemental foods should include yeast, fish liver oil and selenium-containing foods such as garlic or selenium-yeast.
● Use unrefined, cold-pressed oil especially sunflower, sesame or olive oil.

The Problem of Alcohol

Alcohol is a drug too and can cause serious interactions and complications if taken along with other drugs. One of its main effects is to use up resources which the liver needs in order to detoxify drugs. It can also greatly amplify the blanketing mental effects of tranquillizers, sedatives and other psycho-active drugs. The following types of drugs in particular should not be taken with alcohol.

anticoagulants
antidepressants
antidiabetics
anaesthetics
atropine (relaxes internal muscles)
blood pressure lowering drugs
cephamandole (antibiotic)
codeine (reduces pain, stops coughing)
codeine/diphenoxylate (stops diarrhoea)

disulfiram (treats alcoholism)
isoniazid (treats tuberculosis)
metronidazole (treats amoebic and other infections)
narcotics
phenothiazines (treat psychoses and schizophrenia)
phenytoin (treats epilepsy)
sedatives
tranquillizers

Natural Methods of Detoxification

After you have stopped taking drugs, many of the symptoms that might remain such as tinnitus, tiredness, lethargy, headaches, skin problems, digestive problems, allergies, or general feelings of being run-down can be helped by detoxification. This may be quite a long process. Long-term use of many drugs can so impair liver and kidney function that symptoms such as tiredness continue for a year or two afterwards.

Detoxification is accomplished by several procedures which can be guided by naturopathic or holistic practitioners.

Partial Fasting

This should only start after you have stopped the drugs. There are, for example, fruit (grape-juice), raw food, low-calorie, vegan, and macrobiotic brown rice fasts. For best and safest results consult a natural therapist. An excellent fast is the raw food fast. It is a 10-day fast, in which you eat as much as you want of raw vegetables or sprouts in salad, with a little dressing of cold-pressed oil, wheat germ, yeast and cider-vinegar. For 2-3 days you have nothing else whatsoever. After the third day you add any roasted seeds (but not grains), nuts and more fruit, and after the 5th day you add yoghurt. You only go back to cooked foods and cooked grains after 10 days, starting with soups and fish and working slowly up to bread and other wholefoods. Drink only juices, pure water or herb teas.

Do not take vitamin supplements during the fast as you need to be cleaned out of all external chemicals, even fillers in vitamin pills. After that time take a continuous daily supplementation of vitamin C 1,000 mg, vitamin E 200 IU, vitamin A 10,000 units and B complex 100 mg.

Keep to a natural wholefood additive-free diet which will gradually eliminate toxins built up over time and provide essential minerals such as zinc, magnesium, selenium, calcium etc. without the need for further supplements. Aromatic herbs and spices can be a helpful and tasty addition to your cooking.

Ensure a daily couple of cups of 1-2 tablespoons of cider vinegar in hot water with honey to taste, 2-3 cloves of garlic and wheat germ.

Exercise and Sauna Baths

Exercise regularly every day. As it says in the vedic books, it should bring at least three drops of sweat to the brow! Sweating is an important cleansing process and removes drug wastes. Doing it through exercise is more beneficial to the organs than using a sauna. Exercise such as swimming, skiing, football, rowing, running, dancing etc. are all good. Practise deep breathing as you exercise.

But always start exercising gradually. After exercise have a thorough wash, and scrub the skin of your back, torso and stomach. Exercise is an excellent cure for bouts of depression, fatigue or temptation to take further unnecessary drugs or toxins.

Saunas are useful but only when you have stopped taking the medical drugs. You should not take saunas or sudden vigorous exercise with several kinds of drugs, which are, incidentally, also more dangerous in a hot climate. They include antihistamines, β-blockers and other high blood pressure drugs, antidepressants, amphetamines, diuretics, anticoagulants and phenothiazines. Ask your doctor about vigorous exercise and heat if you take these drugs.

Health Farms

It is worth considering health farms or special detoxification centres if you can afford them. They can help to complete the process much more quickly. Some of the tricks of trade are:[20]

● Coolish saunas for 2 hours every day.
● Several spoons of vegetable oil a day to mobilize body fat, vitamin supplementation including high doses of B3 and other B vitamins, and antioxidants.
● Exercise programmes under supervision.
● Hydrotherapy.
● Herbal teas and tisanes to aid elimination and purification (see page 177).

The Vulnerable: The Old and the Young

One of the commonest afflictions of old age is loss of mental function: dottiness. Some of this is irreversible senile dementia. But a proportion may be due to drugs and reversible. It used to be only the bravest of doctors who said *sotto voce* that he has cured some of his confused and demented elderly patients by taking them off all drugs. Now the *British Medical Journal*, in a leading article, has staged that it is surprising that any elderly patient taking drugs should pass a mental test at all. It says that whenever an elderly patient shows signs of mental deterioration drugs should be suspected, and that virtually any drugs can be the culprit.[21]

Elderly people take more drugs because they suffer from more problems, and these drugs interact with each other. They have had more years of accumulated damage from drugs and chemicals and their detoxification machinery is anyway weaker. For example the kidney of an 80-year-old functions at only half the rate of a young adult, or less if there are heart problems, diabetes or drug damage.

Drugs stay around 80% longer in the blood of older people.[17] The average age of people sent to hospital because of severe drug side effects is 60. That makes it all the more surprising that drugs are never tested in the elderly patients nor are efforts made to check how older people react to them.

The drugs which cause most of the hazards are antidepressants, steroid and non-steroid analgesics, anti-inflammatory or antirheumatic drugs, heart drugs, diuretics, sedatives, antidiabetic drugs, tranquillizers and drugs for incontinence. One study found that of a random sample of over-60s, 66% were taking painkillers, 33% drugs for the circulation, 31% laxatives, 30% vitamins, 26% antacids and 22% tranquillizers.[22]

Over-the-counter (OTC) drugs can cause serious nutritional problems in the elderly. Continuous use of antacids causes excess calcium, a lack of phosphorus, overloading with sodium and magnesium and poor absorbtion of vitamins, leading to bone pain and fragility, weakness, nausea, lack of appetite, poor kidney function, and heart problems. Laxatives are addictive and can produce poor absorbtion of vitamins, heart problems through loss of potassium, and bone degeneration. Up to 30% of old people who take aspirin-type drugs may be suffering from stomach damage, (leading to loss of vitamins and nutrients) and kidney damage.[23] Here are some special recommendations to the over 60s:

● Ensure that you are getting the right information from your doctors. An FDA survey found that three quarters of the over 60s were not given any information by their doctor on precautions to take with their medication, and the same number were not told about possible side effects. Make sure you regularly review what drugs you are taking with your doctor, including any over-the-counter drugs, and see if you can dispense with any.
● Try to withdraw from over-the-counter medicines, especially antacids and painkillers. Bulk laxatives such as bran or ispaghula husks are safe; chemical laxatives are not.
● Use daily vitamin supplements and dietary recommendations as described above. Add iron if using painkillers and anti-inflammatory drugs. Add vitamins A, D and folic acid, and vitamin B12, which are the commonest deficiencies in the elderly.
● Take potassium supplements and magnesium-rich food if you are taking diuretics or antacids with bicarbonate, or sodium penicillin, or other sodium-containing drugs.

Mothers and Babies
At the other end of the life span the very young are also extremely vulnerable because their waste-disposal systems are unformed. An

unborn baby may take several times as long to eliminate the drug as the mother and being so tiny becomes loaded with a drug that hardly makes a difference to the mother. This is discussed in Chapter 13 in relation to drugs given to the mother at birth. However *all drugs* taken during pregnancy are a potential risk and their effects on the unborn and the newborn are largely unknown.

Anticoagulants, the antibiotic chloramphenicol, anticancer agents, the anti-infective sulphonamides, lithium, barbiturates, cholesterol-reducing drugs, anti-inflammatory/antirheumatics, anti-gout drugs, thiazide diuretics, tranquillizers, oral contraceptives, corticosteroid, the anti-infective metranidazole, anti-gastric ulcer drugs, diet pills and appetite suppressants, tetracycline antibiotics, bronchial dilators and the anti-epileptic phenytoin, are all drugs that should be avoided at all costs while pregnant or breast feeding. They go through into the milk to a greater or lesser extent.

Make sure you discuss the risks to your unborn or breast-fed baby concerning *any* drugs you are advised to take, and if possible avoid all drugs during this period. In any event breast feed just before you need to take your drug dosage.

Note that stimulant laxatives (cascara, phenolphthalein etc.) should not be taken and that aspirin-type drugs can cause bleeding at delivery.

Be careful of salt and water problems. Simple compounds such as sodium bicarbonate antacids, certain laxatives, or magnesium containing Epsom salts, can produce waterlogging and overweight, and diuretics can cause blood problems in the baby.

Herbs, Homeopathy, and Medical Drugs

It would be convenient if you could take medical drugs to cure diseases and herbal potions to treat the side effects. Unfortunately quite the opposite is true – herbalism and homeopathy cure diseases while medical drugs tend to treat symptoms. In practice if you go to a herbalist seeking advice on dealing with drug side effects he may surprise you by attempting to cure the disease. This does not mean that he can do nothing about drug-induced suffering. But he will regard the use of herbs for symptomatic treatment of drug side effects as a car mechanic would regard a request to put sawdust in a disintegrating gearbox to drown the noise. Any help with side effects will have the aim of taking you off the drugs altogether.

For example a woman in her early 30s went to a herbalist complaining of thrush, a fungal infection in the genital area, while on a long series of courses of antibiotics for a urinary system infection. The thrush is a clear side effect of the antibiotics. The herbalist helped with garlic and a cider-vinegar douche. At the same time he prevented the antibiotics from doing further damage by prescribing acidophilus tablets and live yoghurt three times a day. But this was combined with a strict dietary regime, together with St. John's Wort and other herbs to clear out the infection. The woman came off antibiotics completely at the end of the course she was taking.

Drug side effects create problems for complementary medicine practitioners because they obscure the underlying disease. Drugs suppress the symptom picture of the disease and substitute symptoms of their own. For example complementary medicine would under normal circumstances treat rheumatic problems by working on the circulation and liver to alter the metabolism which creates deposits in the joints. But anti-inflammatory drugs create liver, kidney and digestive system damage which are superimposed on, and hide, the original liver problem. 'The drugs' said one practitioner, 'come between me and the patient.' Steroids are a very serious problem in this repect, and homeopaths especially find that they create such a weird, alien internal world in the body of the patient that the homeopathic approach hardly works.

Nevertheless it is the complementary practitioners job to disentangle all this, and he may do it in a number of ways. He may just treat whichever is bothering the patient most, the disease or the side effects. Or he may treat both at once. He may give supportive treatment while trying to wean the patient off the medical drugs such as painkillers, steroids and anti-inflammatory drugs. Then when they are off the drugs the original disease will be exposed, or flare up, so that it can be treated. The pathway is often flexible depending on each situation and it is a very individual process. No two people will be treated by the same formulae. This whole process takes times. A rule of thumb estimate is a month of treatment for every year of the disease. But the goal of a holistic treatment is a *complete* cure.

Complementary practitioners see a great variety of drug side effect problems. Indeed many will say that they are frustrated by constantly having to deal with doctor-caused ill-health rather than the root of the health problems. Some of the main drug side effects which practitioners constantly meet, and which concern them most, are described here. How practitioners deal with these drugs is described in the following chapters.

Tranquillizers especially benzodiazepines. These present the most frequent problem to practitioners. Patients arrive because of side effects such as tiredness, agitation, digestive problems, hopelessness, sleep disturbances and fear of more serious disease. Some appear in desperation when a new young doctor refuses to continue the endless prescription set up by a previous doctor of the old school. The practitioner will regard such patients as suffering from a dangerous dependency.

Non-steroidal anti-inflammatory drugs. Practitioners see a lot of cases because these drugs create dependency. The inflammations flare up when the drugs are stopped. At the same time they can have profound side effects particularly deterioration of digestion, dizziness and nausea, and kidney damage.

Steroids and other hormones including danazol and the contraceptive pill. Steroids are, in natural healing terms, the most damaging drugs for the entire being. They change the constitution as well as creating the well-known side effects of loss of normal hormone control of the body. Only if steroids have been taken for a short time will there be sufficient gland function left which the practitioner can use as a basis for treatment.

Respiratory drugs for dilation of the airways, and antihistamines. These drugs also create dependency as patients fear they may have asthmatic attacks and spasms if they stop taking them. Withdrawal is assisted by homeopathic potencies, especially if allergic in origin, or by herbal inhalations.

Antibiotics, especially in chronic use, bring a lot of people to complementary medicine, for they feel the original condition is fundamentally untreated and constantly recurring. They also suffer from new infections, such as yeasts or fungus, arriving because of the welcoming conditions created for them by antibiotic usage.

Antidepressants. These have many side effects and patients often come to complementary practitioners with problems. Complementary medicine would treat the underlying mental state by psychotherapy but nerve tonics, dietary treatment and exercise help to restore energy and vitality.

Skin treatments. Steroids, antifungals and other skin treatments for dermatitis and aczema are frequently confronted by therapists because patients are afraid of stopping them. Homeopathic, dietary and herbal treatment will treat the internal roots of the condition. External applications of soothing demulcent and anti-inflammatory herbs such as comfrey, also wheat germ oil, help the symptoms during treatment.

Complementary Medical Aids to Detoxification

The side effects of many drugs continue well after you have ceased to take them. Dietary and naturopathic detoxification methods that we have described above are the main pathways to their elimination and a return to natural health. The process can be helped considerably by other complementary medical techniques. These are some of the methods used.

Bitter-aromatic herbs are often used as liver stimulants. These can be very effective in removing toxins and increasing the flow of bile. The herbs include wormwood, angelica root and myrrh, and can be purchased as tinctures or in ready-prepared 'bitters'. Chinese angelica root has been demonstrated to increase the breakdown of drug substances in the liver.[24]

Blood purifying and liver-repairing herbs strengthen the metabolism and restore a liver damaged by drugs. They include dandelion root, milk thistle, agrimony and echinacea. These herbs clean up the system.

Nutritional herbs. During a clean out herbs should be added to the diet to restore the right balance of minerals in the body, improve absorbtion and elimination, increase vigour and energy and improve sleep. The best herbs for this purpose are alfalfa, parsley or dandelion leaves and kelp. Unlike the other herbs these can be taken without the need for a visit to a herbalist, at a total dose of 25 gm (1 oz) of dried leaf daily, or the equivalent quantity of fresh leaf, or tincture.

Stimulating the kidneys to eliminate toxins can be achieved by several well-known herbs including carrot seed, parsley leaf and seed, or juniper berries. The correct dosages need to be ascertained by a herbalist.

Acupuncture can be very useful for restoring kidney and liver function. Moreover acupuncture is able to make you feel better, lighter and more purposeful, and therefore more able to continue with a self-help detoxification programme. When 20,000 Japanese received partial paralysis as a side effect of the stomach remedy clioquinol (i.e. in Enterovioform), the Japanese government provided them with resources to obtain acupuncture and herbal treatment to speed their return to health.[25]

Homeopathic scrubs are the homeopathic version of blood purifying and eliminative remedies. Typical remedies include nux vomica (6x) with sulphur (x6) or with pulsatilla (6x) depending on the individual constitution. They should be used to remove toxins as part of an overall homeopathic treatment.

Homeopathic Antidoting of Drug Side Effects

Homeopaths select their remedies according to the principle of 'Like-Cures-Like'. The remedy that creates certain symptoms in a healthy person will negate those same symptoms in the sick. If a set of symptoms, such as spasm and diarrhoea during dysentry, are like those produced by a certain poison, e.g. arsenic, then arsenic (in infinitesimal dosage) can be used as a cure. There are different schools of thought in homeopathy, with the classical homeopaths finding the one perfect match or 'simillium' for each person's basic susceptibilities, while others use several homeopathic remedies more eclectically, changing the remedies as the treatment develops.

One discovery, made by both European and Indian homeopaths, is that very small doses of drugs or any poisons will help the body to eliminate the same poison. This hair-of-the-dog phenomenon is hotly contested within homeopathy, but is used by many homeopaths with apparent success against drug side effects. The mechanisms involved are unknown, although they may be a subtle version of the modern use of attenuated or highly diluted vaccines to elicit an immunological reaction in the body. The method is simple. To eliminate a drug from the body and to help deal with its side effects, the homeopath would make a 'potentized' solution of the same drug, at a dilution of many trillions. This would be given to the patient. For example a patient came to a London homeopath after receiving the highly toxic drug roaccutane against acne. The drug had cleared up the acne but just as the acne disappeared side effects appeared – an intense burning in the chest, and all the sweat glands shut down. The young man couldn't wash and couldn't sleep. He was given an antidote to roaccutane made of a high homeopathic dilution of the drug plus basic constitutional remedies to work on the cause of the original acne. Gradually both the basic problem and the side effects cleared up.

One homeopath has made a special study of this subject, which he termed 'tautopathy', as a result of his experience with many patients who have never been fully well since receiving drug treatment for tropical diseases. He saw one woman with a partially cured typhoid plus side effects from chloromycetin treatment. The side effects included burning in the throat, mouth, hands and feet, headache, vertigo, burning eyes, reduced hearing, anaemia and gingivitis. He succeeded to treat some of the symptoms with B vitamins, recognizing that the drug had created a serious deficiency. Most of the symptoms remained, despite treatment with Bryonia and nux-vomica, until he tried a homeopathic dilution of chloromycetin. All the symptoms disappeared within five days and the homeopath could then polish off the residual typhoid.[26]

Homeopaths in the UK vary in their attitude to tautopathy. Some say that such antidoting is bad for the patient in the long run as it further obscures the original condition. Others will use antidotes of tranquillizers, antibiotics, steroids and other drugs to help patients overcome their dependencies, always along with more conventional homeopathic treatment. It has not yet been fully evaluated homeopathically. Of course as far as conventional medicine is concerned, tautopathy is still in the realms of wizardry.

Herbal Self-Help for Specific Drug Side Effects

Taking herbs against drug symptoms is like baling out a leaky boat. As long as you continue with the drugs the herbs cannot achieve any more than a partial palliation, and their effects on health will be wasted. Nevertheless there will be cases where herbs are so needed to relieve drug induced suffering that even in a second-best role of assistant to drug treatment they are valuable. Here are some self-help suggestions for drug symptoms that may occur. You should, however, always take the steps advised on page 164 if you experience drug side effects. These self-help methods must not be substitutes for determined action to stop taking the drugs altogether and achieve healing.

Stomach pains and cramps. One or two drops of peppermint oil or hot peppermint tea several times a day; pains after food can be relieved by the digestive enzymes bromelain (or pineapple juice) and pepsin (or a fresh papaya), and by chewing fennel seeds and aniseeds. Pain from drug attacks on the stomach lining can be helped by slippery elm, comfrey tea and alginates or seaweed products.

Loss of appetite. Aromatic bitters, especially sweet flag, angelica and gentian, taken as a few drops of tincture in water before meals; alfalfa and 50–100 mg B complex taken with meals may help to stimulate appetite.

Nausea and vomiting. Chamomile tea, basil tea or cinnamon and ginger tea can all help. If nausea is combined with gas also use aniseeds or fennel seeds, chewed or as teas.

Constipation. Alder buckthorn, linseed, liquorice and yerba mate tea are all helpful. Enrich the diet with bran, ground linseed or ispaghula husks together with mucilaginous foods like persimmon or figs. Stronger laxatives include senna and cascara.

Diarrhoea. Live yoghurt, especially taken with ispaghula husks, helps. Try slippery elm (put 25g/1 oz in 1.1 litres/2 pints of water and bring to the boil), or cooked blueberries and blackberries and a tea from blackberry root bark or raspberry leaf; enrich the diet with bananas, carob flour and barley.

Insomnia. Teas of hops or valerian or a strong chamomile tea before bedtime help, along with exercise during the day. Vitamin B6 before bedtime can be useful, or obtain the amino acid tryptophan from a practitioner or doctor.

Anxiety/nervousness. Herb teas or tinctures of balm, valerian or passiflora, combined with hawthorn if there are palpitations, will reduce these symptoms.

Skin rashes and dermatitis. Heartsease or golden seal tea externally and once a day internally; use extra Vitamin B complex, E and C with bioflavonoids in the diet; Vitamin E (for itching), calendula and *Aloe vera* creams or applications externally.

Headache. Rosemary and fresh ginger tea, lavender oil or rue to be smelt, peppermint tea and mentholated balms applied to forehead and nape of neck can help, followed by warmth (especially of hands and feet) and relaxation/meditation. Learn the acupressure points for headaches.

Tiredness. Try supplementing your diet with B vitamins and 1 gm vitamin C. Herbal tonics include ginseng with a spare nutritious diet and exercise in the fresh air. Kola nut and Damiana will help.

Cold hands and feet. Rosemary tea or oil or cinnamon oil (2 drops internally) and exercise; also deep relaxation. Use cramp bark, angelica, ginger and lobelia in a tea mixture. Massage with rosemary or mustard oil.

Tinnitus. Treat nutritionally by excellent diet and multivitamins, especially A and C. Deep relaxation helps. Take summer savoury tea and a drop of the oil in the ear.

REFERENCES

1. Office of Health Economics, *Digest of Health Statistics*, London.
2. Boston Collaborative Drug Surveillance Program, *Paediat. Clins. North America,* **19** 117 (1972).
3. Melville, K. A. and Johnson, C. R. *Cured to Death*, Secker and Warburg, London (1982).
4. *J. Am. Med. Assoc.* **144** 1418 (1950); *J. Am. Med. Assoc.* (7 December 1984).
5. Special Commission on Internal Pollution. *J. Am. Med. Assoc.,* **234** 507–9 (1975).
6. Jick, H. *New Eng. J. Med.,* **291** 824–8 (1974).
7. Martin, E. W. *Drug Information J.,* **11** 25–35 (January 1977).
8. Melmon, K. L. *New Eng. J. Med.,* **284** 136–141 (1971).
9. Martin E. *Hazards of Medication*, Lippincott, N.Y. (1971).
10. Lee, B. and Turner, W. *Am. J. Hospital Pharmacy,* **25** 929–932 (1978).
11. *New Scientist,* 8 (2 May 1985).
12. Hermann, F. and Herxheimer, A. In: Soda, T. (ed.), *Drug Induced Sufferings*, Elsevier (1980).
13. *Am. J. Clinical Nutrition,* **39** 691 (1984).
14. Gershoff, and Priem, *Am. J. Clinical Nutrition,* **20** 393 (1967).
15. Roe, D. *Drug Induced Nutritional Deficiencies*, Westport, Conn. Avi (1976); ibid, *Nutrition Reviews,* **42** 141–154 (1984); Oversen, *Drugs,* **18** 278–298 (1979); Mindell E. and Lee W. H. *Vitamin Robbers*, Keats, New Canaan (1983).
16. *Lancet,* **1** 929 (20 April 1985).
17. D'Arcy, *Iatrogenic Diseases*, OUP, Oxford (1976).
18. Nakagawa, S. *et al, Hiroshima J. of Med. Science,* **34** 303–9 (1985).
19. Hsiao *et al, Federation Proceedings,* **34** 742 (1975).
20. Saifer, P. and Zellerbach, M. *Detox*, J. P. Tarcher, Los Angeles (1984).
21. Millard, P. *Brit. Med. J.,* **289** 6452 (27 October 1984).
22. Chien, C. P. *et al, Addict Dis.,* **3** 357–372 (1978).
23. Roe, D. A. *Drugs and Nurition in the Geriatric Patient*, Churchill Livingstone, Edinburgh (1984).
24. Woo, S. W. *et al, Planta medica,* **45** 234–6 (1982).
25. Sonoda, K. and Iijima, N. article in ref. 12.
26. Patel, R. P. *What is Tautopathy?*, Parangot Malekal, Kottoyam (1968).

CHAPTER 10

Drugs For The Mind

Tranquillizers and Tranquillizing Sedatives

Here we are concerned with all drugs of the benzodiazepine class. These include diazepam (e.g. Valium), chlordiazepoxide (e.g. Librium), clorazepate (e.g. Tranxene), lorazepam (e.g. Ativan) and similar tranquillizers; and nitrazepam (e.g. Mogadon), flurazepam (e.g. Dalmane), temazepam (e.g. Euhypnos) and similar sedatives.

Tranquillizers were originally developed to deal with disabling, nail-chewing anxiety, and anxiety connected with medical procedures, for example before operations. They have become the most widely prescribed drugs in the world, with around 15% of the population of the Western world taking them every year.[1] Recent surveys on tranquillizer addiction have shown that:[2]

- patients were given tranquillizers after a first visit to a doctor of less than ten minutes.
- 9 out of 10 were given repeat prescriptions to take them beyond four months.
- 9 out of 10 were not informed of any side effects or that the drugs do not work for long periods.
- 62% had been taking them for more than five years.
- 93% had tried to give up tranquillizers and three out of four succeeded.
- 3½ million people in the UK have taken tranquillizers for more than four months.[3]

Doctors cannot help using tranquillizers as an anodyne for every unspecific pain, grumble or worry that patients bring to the surgery. They have six minutes per patient and tranquillizers are, from their point of view, the perfect complaint stopper. Their effects wear off after a few weeks, for the brain makes a readjustment, and the level of anxiety returns to what it was before.[4] Tranquillizer users then become dependent on them and need to increase the dose, leading to an accelerating addiction beginning after only a couple of weeks of use.[5]

The side effects of tranquillizers recognized by the medical establishment include:

● Anger, rage, hostility, tremulousness, fear, apprehension, insomnia, nightmares and suicidal tendencies.[6] There has been a link between tranquillizers and baby battering.[7] Confusion is common especially in the elderly.
● Depression and, paradoxically, anxiety can be caused by tranquillizers.[8]
● Long-term usage may cause brain damage.[9]
● They can cause drowsiness and confusion, and can make a dangerous combination with alcohol.[10]
● They can cause birth defects and problems for the baby when taken close to the birth or when breast feeding (see Chapter 13).
● There are suggestions (hotly debated) that they might assist the growth and spreading of an existing cancer.[11]
● There may be an increase in the likelihood of diabetes later in life.

'I had started taking Valium for a back problem beginning with 4 mg a day,' writes Barbara Gordon in her book on tranquillizer addiction. 'Now I was up to 30 mg and couldn't get out of the house without taking them.' Her doctor told her they were not addictive. But when she stopped taking them she suffered from a complete mental and physical collapse.[12] Many doctors are unaware how addictive tranquillizers are, despite the US Drug Abuse Warning Network announcing in 1980 that the tranquillizer Valium was the most abused of all drugs, even more than heroin. The most common withdrawal symptoms are: sleep disturbance, anxiety, pains, tremor, headache, nausea, sweating, visual disturbance, fatigue hypersensitivity, depersonalization, psychosis and convulsions. Some of these symptoms occur in one in three of all users, and persist for two weeks or longer.[13]

The tranquillizers protect people from their emotions, and when they are withdrawn the shell is broken '. . . standing at the bus stop and someone shouts at you, you feel as if you have been punched in the stomach,' is how one young man described it. And the symptoms of withdrawal are more profound the more carefully you watch for them. A UK acupuncture clinic issues a leaflet to patients withdrawing from tranquillizers to warn them what to expect. They list over 100 symptoms, from loss of memory, paranoia and disorientation, to urinary and menstrual problems. Needless to say, virtually none of these symptoms is noted in the manufacturer's warnings.

Withdrawing With the Help of Complementary Medicine

If you ask your doctor to withdraw a drug he ought to step down the dosage by one eighth every 2–4 weeks to reach the lowest dose. He may also use different tranquillizers. There is no place in good medical practice for a sudden end to 'mother's little helpers', just as there is no place for doling them out so freely in the first place. Therefore request a step-down withdrawal strategy from your doctor, and some help in locating psychotherapy or counselling.[14] Many people find it hard to step down from the lowest dose to independence, without someone to give them a hand. There are tranquillizer self-help groups that can support you (see Appendix).

Herbal remedies can ease the withdrawal process, bringing you back to your normal self. They must not, however, be regarded as a replacement addiction. The herbs primarily ease tensions in both mind and body, and relieve withdrawal symptoms. One strategy uses the plant tranquillizers scullcap and valerian as main herbs, taken as the chemical tranquillizers are withdrawn. At the same time oat tea may be used to strengthen the nerves, passiflora to prevent palpitations and reduce agitation, tremors etc., motherwort to support the circulation, and pulsatilla or pasque flower to help with nervous exhaustion. Ginseng will reduce stress and restore basic vitality and 'life-force'. The precise treatment programme must be defined on an individual basis. Herbalist David Hoffman recommends 2–4 days on drugs plus herbs, then dropping one sixth of the drug dosage every 4–5 days, working to eliminate symptoms that arise on the way.[15]

Other herbalists rely more on a sedative-tranquillizer mixture, such as passiflora and hops in the evening, along with ginseng to deal with the withdrawal symptoms. One 45-year-old hospital matron had been addicted to valium for years after first taking it because she felt a bit overwrought. She came to a herbalist with irritable bowel/colitis. The practitioner gave her a diet and herbs to clean out the colitis. The valium dependency went over a six-month period with the kind of herbs we have described.

Counselling and constant reassurance and dialogue are an essential part of the treatment. The emotional anaesthesia of tranquillizer use leads to hopelessness and emptiness on withdrawal. Warm supportive connection between the person withdrawing and a practitioner or friend can make the withdrawal much faster. Massage, especially with essential oils, can also help to lift mood and bring back self confidence. The massage returns people to themselves, and oils such as lavender, basil or cinnamon work on the emotional level.

Homeopathy and acupuncture are also useful. A practitioner told us that he uses both techniques to produce symptomless tranquillizer withdrawal. One of his patients was a German physiotherapist who had been taking Valium for 15 years, along with a good deal of alcohol. She had liver problems and was very disturbed. He saw her twice a week for six weeks, using electro-acupuncture to prevent withdrawal symptoms, along with homeopathic sedatives. She was able to stop the tranquillizers, after which she could be referred to a psychotherapist. It was then possible to restore her health with homeopathic constitutional treatment.

Acupuncture can gradually improve mental and physical health to the point where tranquillizers are as unnecessary as earplugs at a string quartet. An acupuncturist told us about a 40-year-old man who suffered from a childhood deformity which gave him a permanent limp. At 21 he had had a nervous breakdown while at work when someone stole his brand-new car, and had been taking medication on and off since then. He had been taking Ativan morning and evening for the last seven years and if he forgot one dose he would get immediate panic attacks and vertigo. He came to the acupuncturist with chest pains which were clearly psychological in origin. The acupuncturist treated him regularly and the pains soon receded. After six months he stopped taking Ativan completely and found the will and energy to begin exercise classes, to change his job and start to re-evaluate his life.

Antidepressants

We are concerned here with both the main types of drug, the tricyclics such as amitriptyline (e.g. Tryptizol), doxepin (e.g. Sinequan), butriptyline (e.g. Evadyne), imipramine (e.g. Tofranil) and others, or monoamine-oxidase inhibitors (MAOIs) such as tranylcypromine (e.g. Parnate), phenelzine (e.g. Nordil) and others.

Antidepressants have more serious side effects than tranquillizers, although dependency is not so widespread. They are nevertheless prescribed too often for problems which are minor and passing or which have their real origin elsewhere than in the mind. For example depression may simply be low vitality derived from poor diet and unhealthy life style, food allergies, low blood sugar, and side effects of other drugs. Antidepressants do help the severely disturbed or those disabled by depression, but the reasons for their use have broadened to include all miserableness.

They are also given to children to stop bedwetting, dressed up in nice-coloured fruit-flavoured syrups. It so happens that most bedwetting is the result of emotional problems and inadequate parental care and the drugs are largely ineffective.[16] That doesn't stop them from being the commonest cause of poisoning in children under five, and they give some children nervousness, insomnia, dizziness, nausea, classroom difficulties and much crying.[17]

For some adults the side effects are more profound than those caused by tranquillizers, including dizziness, drowsiness, dry mouth, blurred vision, headache, constipation, urinary retention, sweating and heart rhythm disturbances. Cases of sudden death of people with weak hearts occur because of these drugs. They can also lead to impotence and obesity. In a recent study of 93 outpatients given these drugs, 31% started to eat excessively and became obese, and 34% had a craving for sugar.[18] Once you start taking them you have to keep going. If you stop taking them abruptly the depression returns with interest, or there are severe withdrawal symptoms. Here are some suggestions.

Drug treatment should be your last resort. Depression can very often be successfully treated by complementary methods, especially where the gloom arises from low vitality. Such methods would include diet, acupuncture, yoga and relaxation, and herbs, which can be combined with psychotherapeutic approaches. The doctor is arguably your last resort, and cannot be regarded as an expert on the causes of, and the solutions to, depression.

Antidepressants react with other substances. The newer tricyclics are better in this respect than the old MAOI antidepressants, which have now been largely superseded because they interacted with substances in cheeses, pickles, wine, yoghurt, liver, yeast extracts, chocolate and pickled herring or anchovies to give high blood pressure. But all antidepressants react with alcohol, street drugs including cocaine, anaesthetics, painkillers and a whole host of other drugs. Since many drugs cause depression as a side effect, never take or accept antidepressants for drug side effects without a thorough evaluation.

Diet and antidepressants. It is important to avoid carbohydrate-rich junk food while on these drugs, as the depression can be made worse. Unfortunately this is the food given to patients in mental institutions taking these drugs. Psychiatric hospitals do not acknowledge any role for the diet in helping patients' problems. They offer diets based on processed refined convenience foods, stimulant drinks and a great deal of sugar, fat, starchy food and dairy products.

Take B vitamins to help cope with drug effects, especially if the diet is poor. The B vitamins concerned are B_1, B_6 and B_{12}.

Magnesium and manganese are important minerals during antidepressant medication. The effectiveness and safety of antidepressants has been linked with the level of these minerals in the blood.[19] Eat magnesium-rich foods, such as nuts, seeds, fish, etc. but do not overdo it.

Tryptophan, D-Phenylalanine and Choline. These are normal dietary factors which, when taken in concentrated form of 1–2 gm, can have antidepressant effects. You may be able to use these preparations as natural antidepressants gradually to replace the drugs. An holistically minded doctor will be able to help you. Tryptophan is obtainable on prescription in the UK, and freely in the US. Choline and phenylalanine are available from nutritionists. D-Phenylalanine (D-PA) is somewhat like acupuncture in its effects on brain hormones, and has been used successfully in research trials to treat depression.[19]

Herbs. There are a number of herbs which can be used as a replacement during and after withdrawal. For example a woman came to see a London herbalist after her GP had taken her off an amitryptiline antidepressant too fast and she had had a strong reaction. The herbalist gave her a diet which was natural-semivegetarian without coffee and tea. He prescribed kola nut, damiana, hyssop and verbena to raise her spirits and bring her successfully through the withdrawal. Ginseng is another herb, which is able to assist vitality during the withdrawal period.

Acupuncture
Acupuncture is very successful at helping people on antidepressants, partly because it acts on the endorphin-producing and emotional centres of the brain, where, according to science, depressive changes are located. It also cleans out after effects of drugs on the internal organs.

Brian Peters saw a lot of hospitals when he was young. He kept on having accidents and was beset by headaches and sinus problems. He was very depressed during adolescence and had been given stronger and stronger medication which he hated, feeling that the drugs were taking his life away. At 18 he was given a combination antidepressant which put him in a state of total panic. He couldn't sleep and felt like a 'crazed junky – wide-eyed and alarmed'. When he tried to stop the drugs every experience became so painful that he soon started them again. He suffered from blinding headaches which mystified migraine clinics, neurosurgeons and hospital doctors but which he eventually found were due to coffee reacting with the drugs. He went on from illness to illness – pancreatitis, orchitis, stomach ulcer, colitis – until he went to a naturopathic osteopath for an injury. This practitioner immediately put him on a strict diet, with written menus, and prescribed herbal compresses. The positive attitude helped Brian to get better though he kept on getting new health problems. He only fully understood them when he saw an acupuncturist who said that his health had been ruined by liver damage created by the antidepressants. The liver was overworking, or 'burning-up' in acupuncture terms. The acupuncturist drained energy from the liver. When I saw Brian later he was fit as a fiddle, young-looking and energetic.

It may seem strange to some that acupuncture can affect your psychological disposition. However depression is not the result of thoughts, more of the state of mind within which thoughts arrive. It is highly susceptible to the flow of life force or, in Chinese terms, the 'ch'i' energy which keeps all your organs well adjusted. Acupuncture can alter the rhythms and function of all the organs of the body including the brain. If depression is like a weak and fuzzy picture on the TV, acupuncture is a bit like adjusting it with a screwdriver. Antidepressive drugs are like hitting it with a hammer. Indeed some of the most subtle psychological side effects of antidepressants – the dislocation of reality and the suppression of the personality – are well treated by the restoration of a sense of balance and wholeness through acupuncture.

The Major Tranquillizers and Antipsychotics

Drugs like chlorpromazine, haloperidol and other phenothiazines used in psychosis and schizophrenia are not likely to be given to patients unless there is a real psychotic episode. On the other hand doctors often do not appreciate how much damage the drugs can do. Indeed there is now a very great deal of evidence that these drugs act essentially by brain damage rather than by the improvement of psychiatric disorders.[21] They are often described as chemical straight-jackets leading to a half-life where patients cannot feel and can hardly talk. If antidepressants bring a hammer to the broken TV, the phenothiazines rip out some of the circuits.

A recent World Mental Health Congress was told that such drugs should be banned: 'More than 25 million patients have suffered irreversible brain damage as a result of these drugs . . . 10 million prescriptions are issued a year in the UK . . . 150 million people worldwide are taking these drugs. . . . Giving people chemicals that cause brain damage to this extent is silly.'[22] This must be the understatement of the year.

The main sign of this brain damage is tardive dyskinesia (t.d.) which is a loss of control over the muscles. It leads to involuntary movements of the tongue and face or jerking and trembling in the entire body. It is mostly irreversible, and comes on during treatment or after the drugs have been withdrawn. It leads to an agonizing choice of continuing to live in suspended animation, or come off the drugs and face t.d. The only clear answer is not to allow these drugs to be given to you or anyone else except in the most extreme situations.

Complementary Medicine

These drugs can have very severe physical side effects: 1 in 200 people have an often fatal drop in their white blood cells, 1 in 70 patients suffer from liver damage, many have hormonal disturbances and eye problems.[23] Mental patients often find it difficult to communicate their symptoms. Therefore it is important to constantly review this medication with the patient and the psychiatrist, and, if possible, to go to see a complementary practitioner to prevent some of these side effects. They can sometimes be helped by the kind of herbal aids mentioned in the last chapter. If you go to a practitioner he will probably request to work with a doctor or psychiatrist in gradually withdrawing from the drugs. Psychotherapy is advisable. Acupuncture would be the best technique to help prevent t.d.

Diet and Supplements

A good diet is essential to protect the organs and minimize damage. Take a natural wholefood diet with plenty of fish and greens. Avoid eating large mouthfuls and eat slowly, as the cough reflex may be depressed. Eat a diet rich in magnesium, manganese and zinc, minerals which are important to normal mental function. These can be obtained from nuts and seeds as described elsewhere. Phenothiazines are reported to block the conversion of riboflavin to its active form in the body, so extra vitamin B_2 should be taken.[24]

Choline is another food factor which may be able to prevent t.d.

The B vitamins can actually be used therapeutically to treat schizophrenia and to prevent t.d. The use of large doses of B vitamins, especially B_1 and B_3, in this way is described as 'orthomolecular psychiatry'.[25] For example over the last 10 years 11,000 patients at the North Nassau Mental Health Center, Manhasset, N.Y. have geen given a vitamin formulation with their drugs. Apparently few of them have developed t.d.[26] The formulation consists of capsules containing ⅓ gm of vitamin C + ⅓ gm of vitamin B_3 + 66 mg pyridoxine + 66 IU vitamin E. Each day 4–12 capsules are taken. These are high doses of the vitamins and should only be taken under supervision of a practitioner.

Narcotic Withdrawal

The main side effect of narcotics is addiction, although there are some transient effects including nausea, constipation, suppression of cough and of breathing and urinary retention. A century ago it was quite fashionable to be addicted to opium. It is estimated that 200,000 people were addicted in the US at that time, and many notables in Europe were quite happily hooked without recognizing it. Some of the addition today is created in hospitals and pain clinics,[27] by premature and excessive use of narcotics.

Of all complementary medical methods acupuncture has achieved the widest recognition for assisting narcotic withdrawal. Narcotics depress the natural opiates, or endorphins, to a level where everything hurts when narcotics are withdrawn. Acupuncture helps to restore these natural opiates. Traditional acupuncturists have long been claiming that withdrawal can be achieved virtually painlessly with manual acupuncture at traditional points. The limelight was stolen by more medical acupuncturists who used ear staples and electroacupuncture to aid withdrawal. However it is now clear that many addicted people go back to drugs unless they have a much more thorough treatment. Today traditional acupuncture is used all over the world for narcotic withdrawal, especially in the Far East, often along with herbal mixtures. Treatment should be given every day for a few days, at ear points which stimulate the detoxification mechanisms and the flow of energy between mind and body. Liver-stimulating points are also used to help the liver break down drug products.[28]

Methadone used to be popular as a replacement during heroin withdrawal on the grounds that it is less severely addictive. However from the acupuncture perspective this is a very unwise strategy. For methadone addiction cannot be easily removed by acupuncture, and causes side effects of kidney damage including waterlogging of tissues, bone pain, insomnia and impotence. It may take months of treatment to overcome methadone addiction but days or weeks to overcome heroin withdrawal.

A very successful model is the Substance Abuse Division of Lincoln Hospital serving the South Bronx ghettos in New York. This clinic treats 80 people a day for addictions, mostly to heroin, on an outpatient basis. They use predominantly manual acupuncture for 2–5 days every morning, and obtain complete relief of withdrawal symptoms. 'Hard-core addicts are usually amazed to discover that daily acupuncture can relieve withdrawal symptoms as reliably as the drugs they use.' After the initial period of daily treatment, occasional acupuncture is given to deal with left-over problems such as depression, and to treat liver acupuncture points to help in cleaning out the body. They find that half of their clients who go through the course remain drug-free for six months. Acupuncture may encourage an emotional balance which helps ex-addicts cope with subsequent life crises without turning back to drugs.[29]

There are other sources of help within complementary medicine, particularly Oriental herbs. A few practitioners in the West can compound herbal 'ch'i' tonics (to stimulate basic vitality) and liver tonics to aid in drug withdrawal. However the proper treatment requires considerable expertise. Two other herbs which are available in the West and have been used for the symptoms of drug withdrawal are passiflora which can deal with agitation, insomnia, pains, cramps and similar symptoms, and gotu kola, which is also relaxing and slightly sedating but at the same time energizes the mind.

REFERENCES

1. Balter, M. *et al*, *New Eng. J. Med.*, **290** 769–74 (1974).
2. Carried out by BBC TV and the National Association of Mental Health, reported in: *Attitudes*, (Summer 1985).
3. MORI Poll, reported in: *Attitudes*, (Summer 1985).
4. Committee on the Review of Medicines, *Brit. Med. J.*, **280** 910–21 (1980).
5. Rawlins, M. and Smith, G. *Brit. Med. J.*, **2** 447 (13/8/1977).
6. Hall, R. *Am. J. Psychiat.*, **129** 738 (1972).
7. Lynch, M. *Brit. Med. J.*, **1** 266 (1975).
8. Morgan, K. and Oswald I. *Brit. Med. J.*, **284** 942 (1982).
9. Lader, M. *et al*, *Psychological Med.*, **14** 203–6 (1984).
10. *FDA Consumer*, (October 1978)
11. Horrobin, D. *Lancet*, 778 (5 May 1979)
12. Gordon, B. *I'm Dancing as Fast as I Can*, Harper & Row, N.Y. (1979).
13. Hallstrom, C. In: Granville and Grossman (eds), *Recent Advances in Clinical Psychiatry*, Churchill Livingstone, Edinburgh (1985).
14. Teare, P. *J. Roy. Coll. Gen. Practitioners*, **34** 258–60 (1984).
15. Hoffman, D. *J. Alt. Med.*, 10 (April 1985)
16. Editorial, *Brit. Med. J.*, 705, (17 March 1979).
17. Weiss, M. *Health Shock*, David & Charles, London (1980).
18. Stein, E. and Stein, S. *J. Am. Geriat. Soc.* **33** 687–92 (1985).
19. *Clinical Psychiatry News* (January 1979).
20. Beckmann, Von H. and Ludolph, E. *Arzneim. Forsch.*, **28** 1203–4 (1978).
21. Breggin, P. *Psychiatric Drugs: Hazards to the Brain*, Springer Verlag (1983).
22. *The Guardian*, 3, (16 July 1985).
23. Shader, R. I. and Di Mascio, H. *Psychotropic Drug Side Effects, Williams and Wilkins, Baltimore (1970).*
24. *New York Times*, C2 (21 July 1981).

25. Hoffer, A. and Walker, M. *Orthomolecular Nutrition*, Keats, New Canaan, CT, (1978).
26. Tzack, C. *J. of IAPM*, **8** 5, 5–8; *J. Alt. Med.*, 14, (August 1985).
27. Portnow, J. M. *Medically Induced Drug Addiction*, *Int. J. Addiction*, **20** 605–11 (1985).
28. Shakur, M. *Am. J. Acup.*, **7** 223–8 (1979).
29. Smith, M. O. *Am. J. Acup.*, **10** 161–3 (1982).

CHAPTER 11

Some Common Medical Drugs

In this chapter we will examine how to deal with the problems that arise from certain classes of medical drugs. We have selected a few of the thousands that doctors can prescribe, which are in common use yet have disturbing side effects.

Antibiotics

The most spectacular results of modern medicine are achieved with the help of antibiotics. There is one thing modern medicine knows through and through, and that is how to use these drugs to kill bacteria in a multitude of different ways. They are apparently so successful that to question their use is heretical.

But their very success is their undoing. For doctors have been prescribing them like sweets for every pain, inflammation, infection or ghost of an infection. This is despite the fact that many infections will go away by themselves relatively quickly, and that many common infections such as colds or influenza are caused by viruses which are not touched by antibiotics. Perhaps family practitioners today are more modest in their antibiotic dispensing than they were 10 years ago. Nevertheless it is still common practice to prescribe antibiotics before a proper diagnosis is made. A study of the way antibiotics were prescribed in hospitals found that in two thirds of the patients given these drugs there was no evidence of a bacterial infection. Yet 1 in 10 received unacceptable side effects.[1] Antibiotics are given automatically to patients undergoing certain types of surgery. Yet a study published in the *Lancet* in 1975 found that infection was three times more frequent in those who had received routine antibiotics than those who had not.[2]

This unnecessary prescribing wouldn't matter if, as used to be supposed, antibiotics attacked only bacteria and left human tissues unharmed. But unfortunately we now know that these drugs are not so harmless. One of their side effects is the disturbance of the friendly bacteria that live in and around the body. The intestine has 1.5 kg/3 lb of bacteria, of around 500 species at any one time, which assist in digestion, metabolism, vitamin production, and elimination of poisons. These are destroyed by antibiotics. The consequences are that septic forms of bacteria and fungus normally held in check begin to take over. These new forms may produce new infections, and they may be resistant to the first antibiotic requiring more exotic and more harmful drugs. The main side effects of antibiotics are as follows:

Digestive problems such as diarrhoea, constipation or nausea can arise from the havoc in the intestines, which are occasionally serious.[3] Elderly people can get life-threatening colitis or diverticulitis from antibiotics.

Tiredness, confusion, headaches, malaise or insomnia can result from the poisons produced by the putrefying bacteria that take over. Antibiotics can also create holes in the wall of the intestines through which poisons can enter the body, leading to allergies. There is also a loss of nutrients resulting from the absence of the helpful bacteria.

Severe allergic shock reactions to antibiotics are rare but are life-threatening.

Specific groups of antibiotics present their special problems. Chloramphenicol can cause fatal aplastic anaemia in 1 in 20,000 cases, yet is still available over the counter in certain countries and over-prescribed in the UK and US. Erythromycin esolate causes liver damage and abdominal pain in 1 in 100 people. It has led to a health authority ban in the US but not in the UK.[5] Sulphonamides and trimethoprim frequently cause rashes and allergic reactions, and can damage the kidney by forming crystals. Sulphonamides can cause a dangerous bone marrow disease and will harm the foetus. Neomycin, gentamycin and similar antibiotics cause deafness in around 1 in 100 people taking them.

Fungus and yeast (candida) infections can occur especially when antibiotics are taken for some time. They attack body surfaces such as intestine, mouth, nose, and vagina. These organisms are normally dormant in the body but are let out of their jail by antibiotics. They cause lasting irritations such as thrush.[6] More seriously they damage the wall of the intestine, letting through intestinal poisons, creating generally poor health, and possibly cancer.[7] Recent research has suggested that this porosity is a cause of food allergies and eczema.[8]

Apart from the direct effects antibiotics prevent the body from properly fighting the disease. The body is left with unhealed residues of disease which may cause much more serious problems later in life. Besides, antibiotics pull the rug out from under the immunity with the result that the disease is more likely to come back.

Avoiding Antibiotics

Someone in reasonable health should be able to get over most infections without the need for antibiotics. You should ensure good nutrition and self-care while healthy. Replace antibiotics by treating common infections with rest, liquids, extra vitamins and the optional additions of natural anti-infective materials such as thyme, garlic, propolis, hyssop, echinacea, golden seal, sage or yarrow.[9] Homeopathy can assist the body to overcome infections and gain immunity.

Long-term antibiotic treatment is much more harmful than a short sharp course. It is also an admission of failure – both of the immunity and the medical treatment. On the other hand chronic infections can damage health and should always be treated in a professional manner. Complementary medicine can often treat chronic infections more successfully and certainly more safely. Therefore, besides the precautions advised in Chapter 2 and 8:

● Check with your doctor if the infection is self-limiting. If so say that you want to treat it without antibiotics. If it is unusual or progressive you should request the 'mildest' antibiotic, or seek help from a competent herbalist or homeopath.
● If your doctor recommends antibiotics ask why he thinks it is a bacterial infection. A laboratory analysis before treatment is often worthwhile to confirm that the antibiotic will actually work. This may help to avoid the frequent hit-and-miss overprescribing.
● Take the antibiotics, if you have to, for the minimum time (but not less than one full course) and then evaluate from the beginning before accepting a repeat course. If the infection comes back consider going elsewhere.

Preventing Antibiotic Side Effects

The thrust of self-help efforts during antibiotic treatment is to attempt to maintain the normal bacterial society in the intestine and on other body surfaces. The more unusual side effects cannot be predicted and prevented. However you can always reduce your chance of being the 1 in 100 case by good nutrition.

Take natural *live* (especially 'Bulgarian') yoghurt three times a day after the antibiotics. This will help to maintain the intestinal bacteria, and stop candida and funguses from taking over.[10] The best way of obtaining this yoghurt is to make it yourself at home with fresh heated milk and a starter culture. Live yoghurt means that it is still fermenting and has not been sterilized. You can also obtain tablets of the beneficial bacteria by themselves. Ask your doctor or your health shop for *Lactobacillus acidophilus* or *Lactobacillus bulgaricus*.

Along with lactobacillus, eat a fibre-rich diet with plenty of green vegetables, carrots, milk products, fish, eggs and whole grains. Do not eat high-protein diets. There are suggestions that a lot of fruit may encourage yeasts, so eat fruit moderately.

At the same time you may need to restore your immunity which is threatened by the antibiotics. *Aloe vera* juice taken internally will help. Herbal blood cleansers such as echinacea, and cider vinegar and honey as a regular drink, are often used.

Garlic and onion help to remove poisons left by the infection which the body cannot clear out because of the antibiotics. Cayenne pepper will help to distribute and sweat out these toxins.

Make sure you take ½ gm vitamin C three times a day while you take antibiotics, Take extra B vitamins to replace those lost in the intestinal chaos. This particularly applies to pantothenic acid and vitamin B_6.[11] Extra vitamin K is needed but can be obtained from fresh green leafy vegetables. Extra vitamin B_2 and folic acid is required with sulphonamides.

Damaging effects on hearing arising from neomycin and similar antibiotics may be preventable by obtaining extra manganese in your diet. This is found in wheat germ and seeds.

Extra vitamin E may help to prevent liver toxicity, produced by tetracyclines, and also the yellowing of children's teeth.[12]

Thrush arising from antibiotics is usually treated by complementary practitioners using a combination of procedures including a douche of thyme tea or cider vinegar to gradually eliminate the fungus. Garlic pessaries also help. A blood cleanser is used, and thyme tea will also work intestinally. The more insidious effects of candidiasis can be treated by holistic practitioners by long-term dietary change combined with anti-yeast and anti-allergic herbs or the mild antifungal medicine nystatin. This is followed by vitamins, especially biotin and B vitamins, and a fibre-rich, low-carbohydrate diet.

In a typical case a patient consulted a complementary practitioner after taking a long course of antibiotics during convalescence after surgery. The therapist responded by testing the blood for candida. The lab report showed yeast-like particles in the blood where none should be. The therapist immediately started the patient on a course of garlic juice, and then *Aloe vera*. Then he repopulated the intestine with *Lactobacillus acidophilus* tablets along with a milk-vegetarian diet. He used herbs, vitamins and a careful exercise and sunlight regime to restore the patient's immunity.

Homeopaths can often eliminate the poisons left over by the antibiotics along with the residues of the infection. One homeopath I spoke to uses potencies of, for example, zinc, sulphur or silica for this purpose, combined with a long-term constitutional treatment.

A strict consistent and excellent diet can often clear up all the residues of antibiotics as well as yeast infections and other side effects, provided it is well managed. We spoke to Andreas, a 27-year-old actress and dancer who suffered from a bladder infection 3½ years ago. She was given antibiotics for 3–4 weeks and then another course for a similar period. She developed yeast infections for which she was given powerful antifungal drugs. Since that time she has had regular bouts both of urinary infections and yeast infections, for which antibiotics were prescribed, yet her physical and mental health worsened. Eventually she saw a gynaecologist for breast cysts who said that the antibiotics were not helping her so she turned to a macrobiotic therapist. He gave her an 'Oriental diagnosis'. He told her that her immunity had been virtually destroyed by the antibiotics, and she was vulnerable to cancer. He put her on a strict macrobiotic diet. She went to cookery classes to learn how to prepare the food. The diet immediately cleared up the yeast and bladder infections. She concluded: 'I gained weight and lost it again, and started thinking and feeling clearer. I have never had an antibiotic since.'

Steroids

Of all drugs steroids are perhaps the greatest villains of the piece. They were introduced after the war as miracle drugs bringing instant relief to arthritics, and it has taken a considerable time for the truth to dawn. The FDA itself now warns the public:

'Many patients quickly reverted to their previous condition when the cortisone treatment ceased. And – even worse – devastating and frightening side effects often accompanied cortisone treatment . . . side effects included insomnia, psychotic behaviour, growth suppression in children, peptic ulcer, delayed wound healing, hyperglycaemia (excessive sugar in the blood), carbohydrate intolerance, muscle weakness, susceptibility to infections and many others. Surgeons reported deaths under general anaesthesia of patients undergoing minor surgery who had been taking cortisone. In addition, cortisone proved to have a habit-forming potential – stopping the drug often brought on withdrawal symptoms . . . Where physician and patient alike had been attracted to the miracle of cortisone they were now repelled . . .'[13]

As if this is not bad enough this list does not include the problems arising from the long term use of steroids such as water logging of the tissues leading to a 'moon face' and heavy body, thin weak bones, diabetes, thin transparent spotty skin, and cataracts. Some of these side effects can occur from cortisone applied to the skin, if it is used repeatedly.

These steroids are normally produced by the adrenal glands to control stress, inflammation, salt and water balance and other important functions. Taking steroids as drugs gradually stops the adrenal glands working. There would be little dispute about the life-saving role of extra steroids in cases where the adrenal glands are diseased or not working, and to treat shock from allergic reactions or serious injuries. However steroids are also used in conditions such as asthma, allergies, rheumatic disorders, eczema and other skin diseases and colitis. In these cases steroids suppress the symptoms of a disease that conventional medicine cannot cure. This puts patients in real danger. For the disease is still there, there are increasing drastic side effects, the steroids cannot be withdrawn without further risks and considerable suffering[14] and, perhaps worst of all, the patient is prevented from seeking a cure for the condition elsewhere.

Doctors know all this but still prescribe steroids since it is irresistibly easy to suppress patient discomforts. And despite complaints from the medical profession, steroid-containing creams continue to be promoted for minor skin irritations. Millions of people are given steroids every year.[15] It is only when the crunch does come, and the patient is badly affected by steroids, that doctors accept defeat. These patients often turn in desperation to complementary medicine. In some cases it is hard for complementary practitioners to help. They cannot conjure up a new adrenal gland. But often there is sufficient adrenal function left to begin restoring health and a skilled complementary practitioner can unwind the tangle of distorted body functions in a remarkable manner, eventually exposing the kernel of the allergy, eczema or asthma and treating that too.

Acupuncture

Acupuncture is potentially valuable in restoring function to degenerated, distorted or damaged organs. It is able to channel energy to the organ in a way somewhat like dredging a blocked irrigation channel so as to provide extra water for a parched crop. In acupuncture terms the damage to the adrenal glands is described as a deficiency of 'kidney yin', or internal energy. Treating the kidney yin points gradually restores the group of functions which it influences, including weak bones, thin skin, poor resistance to disease, waterlogging of the body and lack of energy and libido.

For example a 45-year-old woman came to see an acupuncturist after a pain clinic had given her a course of injections of steroids in her back against severe back pain. The specialists couldn't find any physical cause for this pain, which was unrelieved. But she had gained 13.5 kg/30 lb in weight, had a moon face, perspired constantly, was occasionally incontinent and trembled all the time.

An adrenal test showed that the adrenal glands were hardly working. Her first acupuncture treatment was May 5th at which several points were needled. She felt almost immediate pain relief but it came back after a few hours. She reported the next day that it was the first time she had woken up without pain. Also her hands had stopped trembling. Within two days her perspiration stopped. On May 14th an adrenal test showed that the glands were 80% normal, which is an unusually fast recovery. Treatment continued. She had longer and longer pain-free intervals. By the end of June she had lost most of her extra weight, and by mid July her pain had gone.[16]

One of the acupuncturists I spoke to had weaned several patients off steroids. One patient was on high doses of steroids for systemic lupus erythematosus (SLE). He stepped down the dosage quite quickly with acupuncture and diuretic/liver stimulating herbs such as dandelion. She improved and came off steroids completely in two months. But three months later she fell over backwards while dancing and shattered both her wrists – the bones were very brittle as a result of the steroids. The acupuncturist strengthened her repair processes and her system generally which helped the fractures to mend. He stressed that the bones and the kidney can take up to a year to recover.

A medical study at the Grochow Hospital in Warsaw assessed 36 patients who had been given corticosteroids for bronchial spasms for from two to 24 years. Two out of three were able to stop taking any steroids after an average of 10 months of intermittent acupuncture treatment, and the rest were improved though not cured.[17]

Homeopathy

Homeopaths are divided in their attitude to steroids. Some say they so obscure the symptoms of the disease and the essence of the patient that they can't see the wood for the trees and treatment is impossible. Others say, like the acupuncturists, that as long as some adrenal gland function remains they can build on it. One homeopath described a 9-year-old girl who came from a disturbed family. She had had asthma and eczema since she was a baby and had been on steroids since then. He treated her using various homeopathic preparations – which in her case included pulsatilla, arsenicum, tubercullonium, zinc, and bach flowers. She was able to stop taking steroids internally overnight and slowly worked her way off steroid creams over six months.

We had a letter from a lady who had had eczema since she was a baby and steroid creams since childhood. She noticed her hands becoming thin and transparent but every time she tried to reduce the use of the cream the eczema flared up and stopped her doing any work. She eventually threw out the cream and for three months suffered a great deal. Her hands were so swollen she couldn't use them. Then: 'I heard of a homeopathic practitioner in Leicester. He gave me some Graphites 30 which helped considerably with the swelling. My hands began to heal to the point where I could use them again. The doctor gave me other homeopathic remedies which helped me further . . . my hands are not clear yet, but it's nothing like it was . . . .'

Herbalism

Herbalists will prescribe hormone-stimulating herbs to support the adrenal glands while helping patients to come off the steroids. Extra body water can be drained by herbal diuretics, while herbs such as meadowsweet can prevent the inflammations from flaring up as the steroids are withdrawn. There may be particular promise in Chinese herbs. Certain herb mixtures appear to be as effective as steroids and can be used as a replacement while the steroids are withdrawn. In particular the Chinese herbs bupleurum, hoelen and persica can be used, in various combinations. A study at the Institute of Oriental Medicine in Osaka, Japan investigated 52 patients who had been given long-term steroids for rheumatic, liver and kidney problems. It showed that side effects could be noticeably reduced within three months and they could stop taking steroids after six months, providing they took these Chinese herbs regularly.

Self-help

Extra zinc will help to heal wounds and infections. Vitamin B_6, C and pantothenic acid can help to some extent to protect the adrenal glands and the kidney. Potassium supplements, or potassium rich foods, will protect the heart and other tissues from the effects of water-logging (see section below on diuretics). Eat well to prevent infections, and be careful to prevent injuries and accidents, both of which are harder to get over. In the last analysis, not much can be done while steroids are still being taken. Help is at hand, however, once you begin to taper them off. There is a steroid support society (see Appendix).

Non-Steroid Anti-Inflammatory Drugs (NSAIDs)

Steroids allowed arthritics to throw their sticks away – for a time. The side effects precipitated a rush to find other kinds of drugs useful against rheumatic and arthritic diseases. There is now a proliferation of such drugs, called non-steroid anti-inflammatory drugs (NSAIDs). Many are needed because it is uncertain which one will be effective in which patient. They do not act on the adrenal hormones, like steroids, but on local hormones termed prostaglandins. They are the most widely prescribed of all drug categories. One in seven Americans are being prescribed these drugs and there is a $1 billion market which the drug companies are eager to fill.[18]

As ever the side effects are now emerging, and they are serious. They affect the kidneys by blocking the prostaglandins there, leading to kidney failure, waterlogging, sodium/potassium imbalance in the body and poor general health. The tiny tubes in the kidneys often degenerate, reducing the function of the kidney more or less permanently. If there are pre-existing kidney or heart problems deaths can and do occur from these drugs. There is also a 3–4 times greater risk of kidney cancer.[19] They can also affect the stomach by stripping the lining, which in turn leads to holes through which unwanted materials can filter. This creates allergies.[20]

There are many well-tried natural remedies which can be used as part of an alternative treatment of arthritic and rheumatic diseases. These include black cohosh, blue cohosh, Devil's claw, celery seed, green-lipped mussel and yarrow. There is some support from laboratory studies and in the case of green-lipped mussel from a clinical study for their use in rheumatic conditions.[21] They should be administered in a systematic way by practitioners. Dietary treatment, especially controlled fasts, have also been very successful in reducing symptoms.[22]

Complementary practitioners see many patients taking these drugs and as with steroids treatment must begin with a gradual deliverance from them, substituting natural treatment methods. Here are some of the ways in which side effects can be reduced during this process.

Vitamin E reduces kidney damage caused by the drugs and can prevent scarring there.[23] It should be taken at a dose of about 400 IU per day, but build up to this dose gradually.

The stripping of the stomach lining can be prevented or reduced by slippery elm, comfrey or other soothing 'demulcent' or slippery herbs.

Gamma linolenic acid (GLA) may be a considerable help while dosage of the drugs is being reduced. It is itself of potential benefit to rheumatic or arthritic diseases, for GLA is one of the natural components of the prostaglandin chain that seems to be disturbed or deficient in these diseases. However it cannot express these benefits during drug dosage since the drugs work in the opposite direction. Instead it is quite likely that it can prevent drug side effects by modifying the chaos in the metabolism of prostaglandins created by these drugs.[24] Take GLA while reducing drug dosage, and continue afterwards. It can be obtained as evening primrose oil or blackcurrant seed oil in health shops or chemists.

Aloe vera juice reduces inflammation, accelerates repair and improves the blood supply to wounds, cuts, burns and any tissue damage.[25] There have been many reports that *Aloe vera* also brings relief in inflammations of the intestine, such as colitis, irritable bowel syndrome and stomach pain from drugs. Some initial research suggests that when taken internally it stops allergic reactions created by drugs, yeasts or holes in the stomach lining.[26] You should consider taking *Aloe vera* juice to protect the stomach from the effects of NSAIDs. It can also help with rheumatic diseases as a whole by reducing the inflammation throughout the body, some of which may come from allergic reaction to materials passing into the body from the leaky intestines.[20]

Rheumatic diseases are helped by alkaline diets, low in refined carbohydrates and high in vegetables. Eat only cold-pressed not refined oils. Exclude solanaceous vegetables – tomatoes, aubergines (eggplants) and potatoes. Exclude caffeinated drinks, alcohol, and sugar-containing foods and drinks. Take alfalfa and kelp supplements, vitamin C and B vitamins.

Blood Pressure Drugs

An abundance of advertisements for blood pressure reducing drugs colour the pages of the magazines that doctors read. They may show a family man happily pottering about the house, with the broad hint that life can be wonderfully normal through these drugs. Doctors have been persuaded to prescribe them with abandon to all patients who are diagnosed as having raised blood pressure. That means perhaps 2 million people in the UK, at a cost to the National Health Service of about £120 million per year,[27] and perhaps 20 million people in the United States.

These drugs are of several kinds. The β-blockers block those messages from the nerves to the heart which increase its pumping power. As described on page 158 they can cause asthma and make bronchial problems worse by blocking those nerves as well. Artificially lowered blood pressure may mean dizziness, nausea, cold and cramped hands and feet, depression and tiredness. Then there are drugs which act by expanding blood vessels, which have similar side effects. There are drugs which affect certain hormones acting on the heart. These are potent drugs, though widely used, and cause impotence or sexual problems in one out of two people taking them, besides depression, tiredness, dry mouth and fluid retention.[28] Then there are diuretics, which remove excess body water. Unfortunately they can harm the kidneys, and cause or worsen diabetes. They can produce nausea, stomach and digestive problems, dizziness, headache, tinnitus and bone problems.

To add insult to injury perhaps three quarters of all the patients who have been on these blood pressure lowering drugs do not actually need them. This came to light in the $100 million Mr. Fit study in the US, investigating which factors in the diet encourage heart disease. Nothing much of value emerged from the study which neither proved nor disproved fashionable theories linking cholesterol and cigarettes with heart disease. The only significant finding, which came as a shock to the medical establishment, is that those treated with drugs tended to have a higher death rate than any of the other groups making up this massive study.[29] After much prodding the US National Heart, Lung and Blood Institute finally came out against drugs for raised blood pressure: 'Patients with a diagnosis of mild to moderate hypertension should be encouraged to adopt non-pharmacological approaches as definitive intervention.' That means, don't take drugs; rather, reduce weight, reduce dietary salt, get more exercise and unwind properly, which is, of course, what alternative practitioners have been saying for donkey's years.

A similar 12-year study in the UK run by the Medical Research Council, covering 85,572 'patient-years', found that treatment did not save lives, and did not reduce the risk of heart attacks. Some 15–20% of the patients had side effects including impotence, pre-diabetes and gout, and they withdrew from the study. One stroke was prevented in every 850 people taking the drugs: a niggardly return for such widespread and costly drugging. The medical establishment in the UK also came out against drugs to treat raised blood pressure except in severe cases.[30]

Alternative and Complementary Options
If your doctor recommends these drugs to you, or if you are taking them, here are some suggestions as to what you should do.

Your doctor may not have told you that once you start on these drugs you may be on them for life. Stopping some of the drugs can make you vulnerable to a stroke or heart attack. Make sure you discuss this aspect.

Complementary medicine, particularly naturopathy, herbalism and acupuncture, offers excellent treatment for high blood pressure in its early stages. Progressive relaxation or meditation, a reasonable amount of exercise and dietary control can sort out most mild blood pressure problems. The key herbs are those for relaxing the nerves such as lemon balm or catnip, herbs for sweating such as elderflower or peppermint, those to increase the flow of urine including horsetail and juniper, herbs to reduce fats in the arteries such as garlic, and herbs to open the blood vessels and reduce blood pressure such as limeflower tea, hibiscus tea, and hawthorn. Seek complementary treatment rather than drug treatment for mild to moderate blood pressure problems.

Complementary practitioners will help to protect your heart and blood vessels as you withdraw from high blood pressure drugs. However they acknowledge that once you are on these drugs for some time it is hard to stop taking them. The best strategy would be to go to a complementary practitioner who is also a doctor. Alternatively work with your doctor on a gradual step-down programme, with constant checks along the way, while simultaneously receiving treatment from a complementary practitioner.

Impotence is reversible after stopping the drugs. It can be helped, according to Chinese researchers, by deer horn extracts (pantocrine) available in Chinese shops or supermarkets.

When taking diuretics you need extra B vitamins especially B_6, magnesium, zinc and potassium.[31] Of these only the potassium depletion will be recognized by the average doctor. He may give you potassium tablets. Be wary of them as they can cause stomach ulcers. Instead eat potassium-rich fruit especially apricots, bananas, cherries, grapes, raisins and citrus. The other minerals are obtained from a diet rich in nuts and seeds and green vegetables plus wheat germ, molasses and cider vinegar.

Vitamin E may be able to prevent kidney damage from diuretics.[32] It can also stabilize blood pressure when taken in moderate doses. But high doses of vitamin E taken all at once can *increase* blood pressure, so start with 100 IU and work up to 300 IU per day.

Keep taking supplements of EPA, a polyunsaturated component of certain fish oils. It thins the blood, prevents blood clots and reduces the chances of a heart attack. There is now such a sound backing of research for EPA[33] that it cannot be too long before doctors start prescribing it. As I write this, in December 1986, full page advertisements for EPA are appearing in the magazine *Newsweek*, at a cost to the pharmaceutical industry of $100,000 a time.

Certain side effects of blood pressure drugs such as apathy, depression, lack of concentration, confusion, tremor, muscle weakness and twitches, tingling, cramps, loss of appetite, digestive disturbances and disturbances of heart rhythm may all be due to a lack of magnesium.[34] Diuretics, especially, can drain the body of magnesium. If these symptoms occur take magnesium supplements. Magnesium salts such as magnesium sulphate (Epsom salts) are not well absorbed. However you can now purchase specially designed magnesium supplements containing magnesium aspartate, magnesium citrate or magnesium orotate. Take ½ gm a day.

Certain new drugs for high blood pressure are appearing called calcium blockers. They are supposed to have fewer side effects than the β-blockers, although one is tempted to respond with 'We've heard that one before!' There is evidence that a regime of magnesium supplementation as described above achieves precisely the same results as these new drugs, but more safely and cheaply.[35]

Over-The-Counter (OTC) Painkillers

Those people taking aspirin regularly might be forgiven, when they reach this part of the book, for hoping that I will leave good old aspirin alone! It is true that aspirin and other painkillers are not so drastic as the drugs we have been describing. However aspirin has identical effects on the stomach to the NSAIDs just mentioned. Doctors looking into the stomach can always recognize aspirin users – the stomach lining may be raw and often bleeding. Aspirin may have other effects on the body including a temporary infertility. It slows blood clotting and depletes the body of certain essential vitamins. In the large doses given to arthritis sufferers it can cause stomach ulcers, loss of hearing and tinnitus.

The medical attitude to aspirin has shifted. The DHSS Committee on Safety of Medicines recommends that aspirin should not be given to young children with fever. The British National Formulary also states, 'It is important to advise families that aspirin is not, in the evidence now available, a suitable medicine for children with minor diseases.'

New painkillers are appearing on the market, such as ibuprofen, which are identical to the NSAIDs discussed on page 200. These are strong drugs, as yet untried, and many experts deplore the fact that they are currently on open sale to the public.

Try not to take aspirin and similar drugs automatically to bring down fevers. Fevers rustle up your body defences, increasing antibodies and white blood cells and helping to destroy viruses with the natural virus-killer interferon. If a fever rises, sponge with cold water and keep the head wrapped with cold wet towels instead. Seek medical help if it persists or gets very high.

If you have to use aspirin regularly:

● Take ½ gm of vitamin C three times a day together with B vitamins, especially B_6 and pantothenate. These vitamins help to restore the vitamin losses produced by aspirin. They protect the adrenal glands from being over-stimulated by aspirin and help to protect the kidney. Eat plenty of fruit, green vegetables and milk products to maintain sufficient calcium and potassium.[36]
● Remember that aspirin thins the blood. Do not take it before surgery.

● Take aspirin with milk or food to reduce the effects on the stomach. Taking it with acid drinks such as fruit juices is more harmful to the stomach. Take slippery elm daily to soothe the stomach, as advised in the NSAID section.

● If you feel weak it may be that you are losing quite a lot of blood from taking aspirin, especially if you are elderly. Iron tablets will help.

Paracetamol. The other common painkiller is paracetamol and though this drug does not have destructive effects on the stomach it has worse effects on the liver. The reason for this has been described on page 168. An editorial in the *Lancet* stated that if paracetamol had been discovered today it would never have been allowed on sale without a prescription.[36] For it is deadly in doses very little more than the recommended maximum dose of 4 gm a day. Only 6.3 gm a day has been found to be toxic to the liver,[37] and paracetamol is one of the commonest causes of liver failure. When combined with aspirin it is potentially more toxic than either alone, and may also harm the kidneys.

Don't ever take paracetamol beyond the stated maximum dosage. If you are on a fast, if you drink alcohol regularly, if you have had hepatitis or have a weak liver, don't take any paracetamol.

Vitamin C, E, with sulphur containing amino acids (in egg yolks, garlic and onions) can help to break down paracetamol. However if an overdose is suspected seek hospital treatment with cysteamine immediately, even if there are no symptoms. The symptoms of liver damage appear after 3–4 days when it is too late to do anything about them.

If you have to take a painkiller occasionally aspirin is still safer than paracetamol. But paracetamol is better than certain of the new NSAID anti-inflammatory drugs which may be prescribed as a painkiller such as ibuprofen.

Complementary practitioners should be consulted about any continuous pain if you have no better solution than continuous painkillers. Acupuncture is often very helpful (see Chapter 5). It can treat the pain and 'cool' the stomach 'heated' (i.e. stripped) by painkillers. Complementary therapists with a trained eye may treat side effects of painkillers which you do not at first see, for example a dulled quality in the nervous system leading to a reduced ability to adapt to changes in the climate or personal circumstances.

REFERENCES

1. Moir, D. *et al* In: *Studies in Drug Utilisation*, WHO Regional Office for Europe, Copenhagen (1979).

2. Day, T. K. *Lancet,* **2** 1174 (1975).
3. Midvedt, T. *et al, Microecology and Therapy,* **14** 297 (1984); Berg, R. *Human Intestinal Flora in Health and Disease,* Academic Press, London (1983).
4. Rasic, J. L. and Kurmann, J. A. *Bifidobacteria and Their Role,* Birkhauser Verlag, (1983).
5. Weitz, M. *Health Shock,* David & Charles, London (1980).
6. Miles, M. *et al, J. Am. Med. Assoc.,* **238** 1836 (1977).
7. Bodey, G. *Am. J. Medicine,* **77** (30th October 1984).
8. Jackson, P. *et al, Lancet* (13 June 1981); Peters, T. and Bjarnason, I. In: *Food and The Gut,* Bailliere Tindall (1985).
9. Mills, S. *The Dictionary of Modern Herbalism,* Thorsons, Wellingborough (1986).
10. Conge, G. *et al, Reprod. Nutr. Develop.,* **20 (4A)** 929–38 (1980).
11. Cohen, S. B. *J. Am. Med. Assoc.,* **186** 899 (1963).
12. Wellman, J. S. *et al, Lancet,* **1** 827 (1962).
13. Larkin, T. *FDA Consumer,* (September 1985).
14. Berlinger, F. G. *Postgrad. Med.,* **55** 153–7 (1974).
15. Christy, N. P. (Ed.), *The Human Adrenal Cortex,* 395, Harper, New York (1971).
16. Chen, G. S. *Am. J. of Acupuncture,* **10** 147–53 (1982)
17. Sliwinski, J. and Matusiewicz, R. *Acup. and Electrotherap. Research, Int. J.,* **9** 203–15 (1984).
18. Clive, D. and Stoff, J. *New Eng. J. Med.,* **310** (9) 563–70 (1984).
19. *New Eng. J. Med.,* **313** 23 (1985).
20. Bjarnason, I. *et al, Lancet,* 1171, (24 November 1984).
21. Phillipson, J. D. and Anderson, L. A. *Pharmaceutical J.,* 111 (28 July 1984).
22. Rasmussen, G. G. *Scandinavian J. Rheumatol.,* **88** 53 (1984).
23. Mervyn, L. *et al, Biochem. J.,* **72** 109 (1959).
24. Booyens, J. and Louwrens, C. C. *Medical Hypotheses,* **17** 321–8 (1985); Horrobin, D. F. (ed.), *Clinical Uses of Essential Fatty Acids,* Eden Press, Montreal (1982).
25. Gerstad, G. and Riner, T. D. *Am. J. Pharmacy,* **140** 58 (1968).
26. Bland, J. *J. Alternative Med.,* 8 (June 1985); ibid. *Preventative Medicine,* (March 1985).
27. *The Times,* (11 July 1985).
28. Alexander, W. D. *Brit. Med. J.* **2**, 501 (1975).
29. Kaplan, N. *J. American Medical Assoc.,* **249** 365–7 (1983).
30. Editorial, *Brit. Med. J.,* **290** 322 (1985).
31. *Nutrition Reviews,* **16** 90 (1958).
32. Kushner, J. *Am. J. Clinical Nutr.,* **4** 561 (1956).
33. Woodcock, B. E. *et al, British Medical Journal,* **288** 592–4 (1984).
34. Dyckner, T. and Wester, P. O. *Practical Cardiology,* **10** (15 May 1984).
35. Gaby, A. *Preventive Medicine,* **9** 7 (1984) and *J. Alt. Med.,* 13 (June 1985); *Med. Proc.* **5** 487 (1959).
36. Editorial, *Lancet,* **2** 1189–91 (13 December 1975), quoted in ref. 5.
37. Prescott, L. B. *J. of Pharmacology,* **49** 602 (1973).
38. Manchester, K. L. *et al, British Med. J.,* **1** 1028 (1958).

CHAPTER 12

Risks to the Healthy: Birth

It was a windy Saturday afternoon in March, 1977 when labour began. We were tremendously excited at the prospect of the birth of our first child. The contractions stopped as soon as we got to the hospital, because, as my wife remarked, no one in their right mind would want to be born in such an unfriendly place. Then the farce began. The contractions restarted while I fenced off a series of authoritative suggestions: 'You ought to have an epidural anaesthetic now, it is much more difficult later on.' 'We want to see the baby's heart beat on the screen, don't you too?' which then turned into commands: 'Of course you must have a drip we cannot help you any other way.' I refused the staff. They refused me: 'No, you cannot turn off the fluorescents.'

Then things began to get more intense. Glaring lights, the monitor wheeled in and out, the nurses popping in at regular intervals 'to discuss the epidural'. Then 'We must induce now, you have had long enough' and from a sister: 'Come on, it's Sunday morning.' While we were distracted by irritating medical debates the birth was induced. The contractions stormed. My wife screamed. 'Don't shout, you are disturbing others – you are not alone here you know!' The baby was taking its own time. The midwife came in: 'What? Still at it? If you haven't had the baby in five minutes we will use forceps.' 'Push!' 'I'm not ready.' 'Push!' Under threat, in pain, the baby was born.

We were all fine, but depressed at the loss of our birth.

'Imagine yourselves,' obstetricians at the 3rd International Congress of Obstetrics were asked, 'about to embark on a perilous, difficult, physical effort upon which your entire future depends . . . you have two belts firmly strapped around your middle with wires passed to your genital organs. A drip is in your arm. Now you can no longer move about or change position. Machinery is standing between you and your friends who were helping you before.' Even obstetricians have become alarmed at the absurd degree to which medicine has made births more difficult and sometimes more dangerous.

For example a study by Professor Mehl at the University of

Wisconsin of 2,000 births compared those born at home with those at hospital. There were 30 birth injuries at hospital, none at home, 52 babies needed resuscitation in hospital, only 14 at home, and six children had neurological damage in hospital and only one at home. Of course one might expect that more high-risk cases go to hospital, and there should be more still births there, but birth injuries are created at the birth, and hospitals are meant to prevent them, not create them.

Consider the mortality statistics. There are 18–22 infant deaths per 1,000 born in the US which offers the most medicalized births in the world. Yet Holland, where half of all births are at home attended by midwives only, has only 11–14 infant deaths per 1,000. One mother dies in Britain for every 6,600 births, while only one mother in 25,000 dies in Holland. The Head of Obstetrics at one of Amsterdam's main hospitals commented that in his experience only 3–5% of all births need a doctor in attendance.[1]

The baby suffers from medical interference in a multitude of ways, and only a few experts really understand how to read the signs. The editor of *Birth and Family Journal* writes: 'The bright-eyed, quiet, attentive newborn, who is the product of a birth in which the mother was relaxed, constantly supported, fully mobile, unmedicated, delivered gently and quietly . . . is not recognized in hospital obstetrics. Most nurses and obstetricians actually believe we are talking nonsense when we talk about them.' The experts expect, instead, 'A sleepy neonate, one who does not focus the eyes or follow objects and mimic faces, one who feels poorly, is hard to "contain" or comfort and has fewer or no periods of "quiet alert" state.'[2]

Throughout this book we have been talking about risks and benefits in relation to medical treatment that you are considering for an illness. Birth is different because it is not an illness, and any medical side effects are wreaked mostly on two healthy and innocent people, who are trying to carry out a natural, powerful and ultimately fulfilling act. This makes the side effects all the more serious. It is true that there is a very small percentage of high-risk birth cases, and birth is a risky moment in our lifespan. This is the expressed reason for all the obstetric procedures and paraphernalia. But in order to justify itself and in an excess of zeal this birth apparatus has encompassed every birth, normal or not.

This is particularly true in the US, where one paediatrician complained: 'Almost every stage of obstetric practice in the hospital is part of the mechanism that enables the doctor to create his own pathology. Once he has created the pathology he has his excuse to intervene.'[3]

How can we avoid these problems? Where does one begin? The

problem with advice to parents is that as every life is different, every birth is different. The whole pregnancy and birth process is bound up with feelings, psychology and inclination. Furthermore there is no point in advising mothers of the consequences of birth procedures. The procedures will be carried out anyway and the mother will now add guilt to her other problems. Are there certain key moments of the birth, points of decision, where some help in weighing pros and cons would be valuable?

I asked this question of a Lamaze teacher who has been teaching teachers of natural childbirth for 12 years. She confessed to being quite depressed.

'Most of my teaching is wasted because the mother cannot resist the onslaught of medicine with its apparently superior knowledge.'

There are no decision points because the mother's confidence in herself is taken from the beginning.

'You can learn all you want, argue, ask questions, you may even win a skirmish, but you will lose the battle. Your will is removed right from the prenatal checkups. Your baby is tested with equipment, you are introduced to pathology and the continuous feeling of risk: something may be wrong. The doctor makes out he knows more about you than you know about yourself. No one will trust the mother right from the beginning, and soon she no longer trusts herself. From then on the mother becomes more or less a patient and it is only natural that she really is a patient at the birth. You ask me which are the adverse effects. The whole thing is an adverse effect.'

Obviously the answer would be to have home births. But this advice is unrealistic in most countries. Midwives who work in the community are few and far between in the UK. The male-dominated medical profession has, indeed, mounted a campaign over the years to take birth out of the home and the hands of the community midwives, and place it under its control in the hospital. Almost 100% of births are in hospital in the US and midwifery is more or less forbidden outside them.

So we will assume you are having a hospital birth and seek to minimize medical manipulations and their side effects. First we have to understand what these effects are. But in case reading the sagas below makes you despondent, let me say that recently many hospitals have changed and offer mothers a family-centred birth, with more choices. We went to the same hospital for the birth of our second child as our first. This time we requested beforehand to be left completely alone, which they respected. We went there at first light and were home with the baby for breakfast.

The Obstetric Gauntlet

Ultrasound

This is one of the first medical items on the birth menu. It is now used almost universally during the antenatal period to check rate of growth, due date, normal structure and foetal heartbeat, which it does using high-frequency sound waves in a manner similar to radar. There are no reports or evidence of harmful effects in the West. However there have been unconfirmed reports of abnormalities of the foetus from research in Japan and doctors there apparently do not use it in the first three months of pregnancy.[4] It is probably reasonably safe, but only use it if you need to.

Shaving and Enemas

These are no longer routine but you may still meet them. They are widely acknowledged to be unnecessary indignities (see Chapter 6).

The Birth Position

Lying flat on your back. How can this relaxing posture be called a medical side effect? It certainly can, because there are certain things that you should not do lying immobile on your back, namely eating, defecating, drinking and having babies. Traditionally midwives were well aware of this and a major item of their equipment was the birthing stool. Evidence has been accumulating since early this century that squatting or sitting opens the pelvis, increases pressure in the abdomen, recruits gravity to help you deliver, and eases contractions.[5]

Yet medicine has turned the mother into a supine patient, because medical procedures such as drips, electronic foetal monitoring, episiotomy and forceps, all require immobility. I remember being told by a rather cynical Oxford obstetrician a few years ago, how immigrant Pakistani women struggled bravely to deliver their children lying on a bed, too timid to protest to the professional males around them, until *in extremis*, at the last moment, they leaped off, pulling tubes and medical pieces with them, to deliver healthy babies squatting in the corner of the delivery room 'like frightened rabbits'.

The fact is that while the mother is supine, the weight of the uterus and foetus depresses a main artery to the placenta. When the mother changes from sitting to lying position foetal oxygen supply drops noticeably within two minutes. Strapping the mother down to measure foetal heart rate can produce abnormalities in foetal heart rate!

At the same time it harms the mother's blood pressure, decreases the contractions, inhibits the mother's efforts to push her baby out, inhibits the natural expulsion of the placenta, and increases the need for forceps, induction, episiotomy and Caesareans.[6]

The sitting position is used in Holland where only 4% of births require forceps, compared to the US where forceps are used 10 times more frequently. Comparing flat-on-back versus sitting-and-moving births shows that the latter are up to one third shorter with less pain and complications. Sitting births are beginning to be used more frequently in the UK.

The Artificial Induction and Stimulation of Birth

The mother is blessed with a complex natural timing mechanism to bring on labour when the baby is ready. The womb contractions that eject the baby are controlled by a hormone from the brain, oxytocin, as well as others in the uterus itself. Artificial oxytocin, suntocin, is used in hospital to stimulate contractions. It is given in a carefully measured dose by continuous drip into a vein, and the doctor will also artificially break the waters.

There are certain medical situations where induction is necessary. These include toxaemia, diabetes, a very late birth (over two weeks past the expected date of delivery) or foetal distress. These would account for 3% of all births. Instead around 20% of births are induced or stimulated. It became a matter of convenience for the doctors to have the babies before tea and reduce the amount of night work. A storm of protest in recent years resulted in a directive from the FDA that induction created risks for the mother and child and should not be used for purposes of convenience. This has helped to modify UK hospital practice.

So what are the problems with induction? The obvious one is that if the baby is not ready, and has to be kicked out by the obstetrician, it may be premature. 'There will inevitably be a proportion of cases in which an error in the dating of gestation results in a premature child who may die or suffer irreparable damage in the neonatal period' writes the *Lancet*.[7]

Induction produces a 'tumultuous birth' – extremely strong and frequent contractions which are painful to the mother. They make the mother lose control of the birth and the baby can be damaged by the strong contractions without protective waters around it. The blood supply to the baby is reduced and the umbilical cord more likely to be compressed or twisted.[8] If the dosage of hormone is a bit too high, a whole collection of tears, ruptures and haemorrhages could result.[9]

These problems mean that induction is usually the open door to a trail of further medical procedures. For example painkilling medication is almost universal in induced births, 6–7 times more frequent than in an uninduced birth. Forceps are more likely and real or false alarms on the monitor lead to increased Caesareans.

There is now good evidence that induction of labour may cause jaundice, which affects some 10% of babies at birth, possibly by disturbing the baby's hormone system.[10] Other authorities suggest that it is the glucose drip itself, routinely given to mothers, that causes the jaundice.[11] We discuss how to avoid unnecessary induction below.

Abdominal Foetal Electrocardiograph (UK) and Electronic Foetal Monitoring (US)

These machines, which we will call EFM for short, are electronic versions of the stethoscope. They record the baby's heartbeat on a screen. They are usually strapped around the mother's abdomen, or attached to the scalp of the unborn baby with a small screw after rupture of the membranes.

As with much medical monitoring equipment it is used as a substitute for personal care. The National Perinatal Epidemiology Unit at Oxford has found that mothers were left alone more when EFM was used rather than the traditional midwife's ear trumpet. The mothers felt more deprived of the reassurance of good nursing care.[12] The machine also tends to be used as a substitute for knowledge, intuition and experience. They are not particularly reliable and it may take no more than a mother's tummy-rumble to send her off to a Caesarean, at least with inexperienced doctors. Caesareans are 3–4 times more frequent in monitored births. This may also be because monitoring prevents the mother from moving about.[13]

The definitive Dublin Study, at the National Maternity Hospital in Dublin, examined no less than 12,964 births. They could not find any difference in survival and health of the baby as a result of using EFM compared with the ear trumpet.[14] It is only useful in a few cases where, in skilful hands, it can actually prevent unnecessary Caesareans.

Painkillers, Anaesthetics, and Tranquillizers

At the beginning of your labour someone will ask you what anaesthetic you want. It is assumed you will have one. It is true that pain can be intolerable to a mother in childbirth, and as it is within the power of modern medical technology to alleviate it completely, you should be given the option of a painless childbirth. But it is not a something-for-nothing deal. There are costs, especially to the baby, which you are not always told about.

During pregnancy the body's own painkillers (endorphins) accumulate in the brain and lead to a natural analgesia and a very pleasurable 'high' – the peak experience of childbirth.[15] These endorphins may also help to initiate milk secretion and the first loving connection between mother and child.[16] However anxiety, stress, fear, and loss of confidence all reduce endorphins and increase pain sensitivity. These are the states of mind encouraged by medical obstetric interference, and obviously the interference itself may require anaesthesia.

Many more mothers could have a drug-free birth if they prepared themselves beforehand and were given the emotional support to pass through the experience using their own resources.[15] As one mother writes:

'I felt that I could actually manage my response to the strangeness, the unaccustomed unfamiliar wrench of contractions, and that in some way altered the concept of labour being "painful". On reflection, pain does not transpose to memory. Just as well. But it did exist and I did have to handle it. Drugs did not help at all. Some sort of self-control did. Perhaps it was partially pride and exhilaration at being able to handle all those raging feelings which acted as a kind of natural drug?'[1]

The drugs are:

1. Narcotics, close to morphine, such as Pethidine or Meperidine
2. Tranquillizers to reduce tension and the side effects of narcotics
3. Regional anaesthetics injected into the spine, in particular epidural or spinal blocks
4. Gaseous painrelievers particularly Entonox (nitrous oxide and oxygen)
5. Total anaesthetics in the case of a Caesarean.

For the mother, such drugs produce a dozy and out-of-touch state that makes it more difficult to manage the birth, which is more likely to be managed by others: 'It could make the difference between a nightmarish haze and an exalting – if not effortless! – experience.'[1] As epidural anaesthesia stops most feeling below the waist, you cannot push the baby with the contractions. The birth therefore takes longer, and there is more chance of a forceps delivery and tearing.

All drugs cross the placenta and affect the baby. Not only is the baby very sensitive to drugs, but it is receiving the same dose as the mother although it is one twentieth of the weight. The birth is also the time when the baby's brain is developing at its fastest. The drugs act on the respiratory centres of the brain and the baby may be deprived of oxygen at the most critical moment of its life.[17] The infants are born sluggish and unresponsive. They may not cry or breathe so soon and may suffer actual foetal distress leading to emergency care. There is a delay in growth rate.[18] Psychologically, children born of drugged mothers show less attention, orientation and sharpness.[19,20] The baby and mother seem to have less intimate contact,[21] and psychologists can notice these effects up to one year later.

Professor Yvonne Brackbill and Dr Sarah Broman collected all the available studies on this subject and threw them at the FDA. Every study reported immediate harmful effects of birth drugs on the development of the newborn, and some showed effects noticeable years afterwards. The FDA agreed to warn doctors.[22,23] Epidurals were found to be less harmful than narcotics to the psychological development and intelligence of the baby, but they certainly did affect the respiration and heart rate. Gaseous pain relievers appear to be much safer than the above drugs.

Tranquillizers taken by the mother at birth, are disastrous for a newborn baby. The baby does not feed properly, and often has to be tube fed. It can hardly use its muscles, and has low scores of infant intelligence. The effects last for at least a week after the birth as the baby cannot seem to get rid of the drug properly. Tranquillizers do not relieve pain and there should be no reason for a mother to go anywhere near one.[24]

Caesarean Section

Julius Caesar is supposed to have been born by surgery, so the modern technique of opening the mother's abdomen and removing the baby is called Caesarean section. It might have been so named because of the trouble the Caesars gave their mothers, for Caesarean section is an obstetric extreme. You are usually given a total anaesthetic as for any major surgery, then shaved and painted with antiseptic. With an intravenous drip and a bladder catheter you are wheeled into the operating theatre. The abdomen and the uterus are opened, and the baby removed. It takes 5–10 minutes, and then 45 minutes of stitching. You start walking within 24 hours and if all goes well you should be out of the hospital after a week.

There are considerable risks in Caesareans, despite the blithe assertion of the classical medical text on childbirth, *Williams Obstetrics*, that 'there are virtually no contraindications to Caesarean section.'[18]

The most common side effect – the one least considered by the medical world – is depression. The majority of mothers report a feeling of helplessness, depression, failure and perhaps some guilt because they had no active part in the delivery.[15] The mother and baby are separated at the crucial moments. The anaesthetics and subsequent painkillers have the side effects we have just described and may create problems with breastfeeding.

There is quite a lot of pain after a Caesarean and infections are also very common; they affect four out of 10 mothers. Many mothers haemorrhage and 10% require blood transfusions, which bears a limited risk. The death rate for mothers is up to 20 times greater than that of normal births. In the UK it is 1 in 1,000, half of which are from anaesthesia.[25]

As far as the infant is concerned many of the problems occur because it is often taken from the womb before it is ready. This, together with the Caesarean itself, may give the babies a lung problem called respiratory distress syndrome.[26]

These risks are sometimes worth taking, in order to save the life of the child or even the mother. Such cases include:

● Placenta previa: if the placenta covers the cervix or comes in front of the baby.
● Cord prolapse: if the cord comes down the birth canal before the baby.
● Severe toxaemia: if the mother has high blood pressure and inability to clear waterlogged tissues.
● Virus infections of certain kinds.
● Separation of the placenta.
● Diabetes.
● Foetal distress in real cases of lack of oxygen reaching the baby.
● Cephalopelvic disproportion (not in all cases – see p. 221), where the head of the baby is much too large for the pelvis.
● Abnormal position (not in all cases – see p. 220): usually the breech presentation in which the baby is positioned buttocks first.

Now these reasons should at the most amount to 5% of all births. In fact there was a time when if an obstetrician had a record as having more than this rate of Caesareans, his colleagues would tease him. Today the Caesarean rate is 2–3 times greater in Europe and four times in the US. This is partly the consequence of all the other medical steps in birth. As Dr Mendelsohn wryly remarks: 'If immobilisation of the mother, artificial rupture of the membranes, drugs, induction and foetal monitoring all fail to produce a convincing symptom as an excuse for a Caesarean, the doctor always has one card up his sleeve. He can shake his head sadly and blame the victim by telling the mother that her pelvis is too small to permit the birth of her child.'[3]

There are other non-reasons for Caesareans, including the fact that it is fashionable (just as tonsillectomy once was), that obstetricians feel they may be sued if they do not do everything, that it increases obstetricians' incomes, and, more to the point, that obstetricians, like all doctors, have a lack of training and experience in *normality*.

There is an assumption among obstetricians that once a Caesarean always a Caesarean. This also produces a crop of unnecessary Caesareans because the actual likelihood of harm to the mother from a vaginal birth after a Caesarean is very small, and is actually less risky than the Caesarean itself.[28] At least three quarters of all women who have had one Caesarean can be recommended to have a normal birth.[27,29]

The fact that all these Caesareans are unnecessary is proved by the fact that, apart from the 5% of real cases, the extra Caesareans do not produce healthier babies.[30] This is even true for those babies breech born: 'Even among those infants with a breech presentation, a group believed to particularly benefit from Caesarean births, the data failed to show any mortality reduction,' concluded one authoritative assessment.[31]

Thankfully there are signs that this trend is turning tail. In 1980 the National Institutes of Health issued new guidelines telling doctors that vaginal birth for women who have had a previous section is safer than another section. It also stated that women should be encouraged to walk about if contractions are not strong enough. However you can easily still be faced with an unnecessary Caesarean for the above reasons. Obstetric practices die hard.

Episiotomy

The birth is nearly over, and the doctor comes to cut your perineal region, because of another dogma that a clean surgical cut is more easily repaired than a ragged tear. It is thought to ease the passage of the baby's head out of the birth canal. It is the second most common surgical procedure in the Western world. Despite this there is little evidence that it actually does prevent tears, and a study of 17,000 births has found that it does not matter to the baby whether it takes a short or a long time to travel down the birth canal.[32] The *British Medical Journal* reported that quite a few mothers will have no tears at all, and those with tears have less pain than those with episiotomies. Major tearing only happened in those who had episiotomies![33] Besides, episiotomies can lead to scars, wound infection, and pain on intercourse for several months (one in five women). Women with tears resume sex before those who have episiotomies.[34]

The episiotomy seems to be another surgical fashion:

'Sedated, feet in stirrups attached to an intravenous fluid bag and a battery of monitors, the woman in labour is set up so well for surgery, an operation had to be invented so the scene wouldn't go to waste. Enter the episiotomy.'[35]

The Special Care Unit

If the baby has any problems or is premature it may be whisked off to a special care baby unit (SCBU) in the UK or neonatal intensive care unit (NICU) in the US. In some hospitals one in four or one in five babies are incarcerated in these twilight zones, at risk from infections, enclosed in incubators and attached to machines.

There is no doubt that in serious cases of prematurity or foetal distress the special care unit can save lives. Yet if there is no local special care unit the babies are usually not sent, and they are none the worse for it.[36] Only 15% of home birth underweight babies are sent to the units, compared with 70% of those in obstetric wards of hospitals, with no difference in result.[37]

Martin Richards, head of the medical psychology unit of the University of Cambridge, comments that babies are sent to these units because of attitudes of the staff, because of the pressure of administrators ('Why haven't you got your beds full?') and because of equipment salesmen.[36] In fact UNICEF reports that the world-famous obstetrician Dr Caldeyro-Barcia packs premature babies under their mothers' clothes next to her skin, with ample breast milk, and saves 90% of babies from 1–1.5 kg/2¼–3 lb, a statistic much better than that of the special care units.

How To Reduce Medical Interference in Your Childbirth

Preparation

You should do your best to assume that your birth will be a normal, natural and fulfilling experience. Just as doctors did not take over the intercourse which conceived the baby, there is no reason why they should take over your delivery of the baby which was conceived. It is essentially a personal, private experience, involving you and your partner or helper only. Why should you let it out of your hands?

Your guardians are your faith in yourself, your sense of wonder, and your relationships with your partner and your baby. Even if it seems inconceivable that this little pelvis will accept the baby, that these breasts will actually produce milk, that this mind could ever suffer the pain of childbirth, you can assume that your body will rise to the occasion.

Your relationships help during the preparation for birth so that you do not feel alone while having to make critical decisions affecting you and the baby. However they really count during the birth itself. For resignation to medical procedures is often a frustrated cry for help during a difficult moment, directed towards the wrong people.

The pregnancy is the time to get informed on the birth. There are several good books on natural childbirth, which are described in reference 38. You should read as much as you can. Go to childbirth preparation groups in your area (see Appendix). Make sure that the classes prepare you for a possible medical intervention in birth. The hospital routines and interventions create distractions, anxieties and confusions which tend to chase natural childbirth education out of the window.

Which hospital is the best? You should generally look for the best person rather than the best place. However in the UK you would be recommended to go to a small GP unit, staffed by general practitioners, rather than an obstetric unit of a larger hospital under the care of a specialist. The GP units produce less complications and you will benefit from your existing connection with your general practitioner – and so will he or she. Make sure too that the hospital will allow you to have your baby with you as much as you wish.

You may be tempted to go to private medical care, since you will be given greater freedom and more personal attention and comfort. But be warned. Private medicine sells medical care, which is just what you are trying to avoid. There tends to be more medical interference.

In the US the best places are also out-of-hospital birthing centres, or alternative birth centres. Failing that, seek a hospital with a family birthing room.

Of course hospitals and birth centres change, depending on the attitude and personality of the obstetricians and doctors. You may find an enlightened obstetrician even in the biggest hospital, with an excellent reputation for the encouragement of natural birth. This information is usually available from local childbirth groups. Choose a doctor with a reputation for assisting home births and normal births, and without a reputation for Caesareans. He should preferably be a family physician or a general practitioner, if not, an obstetrician, and lastly a gynaecologist.

Here are some questions you should ask:

● Does he support and agree with self-sufficient and natural birth?
● Does he encourage fathers' participation and is this encouraged by the hospital where he works?
● Is he prepared not to use electronic monitoring devices unless there are problems?
● Does he give the labour the time it needs, within reason?
● Does he encourage mothers not to have epidural or spinal anaesthesia unless it is absolutely necessary?
● Is he experienced at vaginal delivery for a breech baby?

● Will he be prepared to allow the mother to go into labour even though a Caesarean is probable afterwards?
● Does he give the baby to the mother straight after birth?

You can also prepare during the pregnancy for alternatives to painkilling drugs. The childbirth classes will teach breathing and relaxation, which do help a lot. You can make a connection with an acupuncturist who will give you obstetric acupuncture (see page 223) in case you need it. Make sure you have a nourishing and natural diet during pregnancy. This helps to reduce unexpected complications.

The High-risk Pregnancy

Most of the difficult births are known about beforehand. So supposing you are in a high-risk category and can perhaps expect a difficult birth or Caesarean. What should you do to minimize the medical side effects?

Breech Birth

Only 3–4% of pregnancies result in a breech presentation, in which the baby attempts to come out bottom or feet first. It is a common reason for a Caesarean, but there are no hard and fast rules and successful vaginal birth is possible depending on the size and shape of the pelvis and cervix, the weight of the baby, how the labour is going, and the kind of breech position. The key lies with the doctor or obstetrician. Many are not experienced in the vaginal delivery of breech birth. However you can and should find others who deliver healthy babies in the breech position without extra risk, after a careful evaluation of each case.[40] The birth must not be induced.

The breech can sometimes be turned by postural exercise beginning at seven months. This involves relaxing for 10 minutes twice a day on a hard surface with knees bent, and pelvis raised about 30 cm/12 in by a pillow. Some midwives and obstetricians can also turn the baby from outside, but they must know what they are doing.[41]

Acupuncture can help breech babies to turn. In China this is very frequently used and there are reports of an 80% success rate using a very simple procedure. It often involves 'moxa', that is burning little cones of a certain leaf of a plant over an acupuncture point. Here is such a case described by a woman in London who wanted a home birth:

'At 38 weeks gestation my second baby was still in breech position and my obstetrician who felt sure that the baby would not turn, made no attempt to turn it himself. Not willing to take unnecessary chances, and knowing that a breech baby meant hospital birth, I went with my midwife to see an acupuncturist. Using moxa on my little toes on alternate feet was, to my mind, a little bizarre; but as he applied the 6th cone and I felt the heat from it, I simultaneously felt a sort of gravitational pull towards the baby. To everyone's amazement the baby's head moved from the right side of my stomach over to the left. At the end of the treatment, the midwife put her hand on my tummy and gently moved the baby a little further round. I then felt a most peculiar sensation as the baby kicked himself the rest of the way round so that his head was in the right position. The same night the head engaged. I was delighted.'

Small Pelvis

The diagnosis of 'cephalopelvic disproportion' is an excuse for many unnecessary Caesareans. Therefore if you are given this diagnosis you should seek another opinion from a doctor with a long experience of normal delivery. In many cases further tests such as ultrasound and a detailed examination just before birth will show that adjustments are being made by both the baby's head and the pelvic structure to allow a normal delivery. In any event you should be allowed to go into labour naturally even if a Caesarean is thought necessary by your second-opinion doctor.

Vaginal Birth After a Caesarean

It is hard enough in our culture for women to trust themselves and to be at one with the birth experience. For a second birth after a Caesarean it is even harder, since their bodies did not appear to work properly the first time. Failed expectations, doubts and fears are more problematic to a second vaginal birth after a Caesarean than the medical risks themselves.

The first task is to understand fully why the first Caesarean happened. In a good many cases it will have been unnecessary, and in other cases, such as breech birth, exceptional. You can start again, this time with better information and a better doctor. Choose one who will be happy to escort you through a vaginal second birth. Many will not, or will at least place many medical restrictions on such an event.

If you try to deliver normally, and there are further problems and a second Caesarean is necessary, at least you know you have tried. There may be one in five cases where a Caesarean becomes necessary again, usually because of rupture of the uterine scar, but this is not dangerous.[42]

The best chances of success are:

● If the reasons for your previous Caesarean are absent.
● If you have a normal pregnancy.

● If you have had a previous vaginal birth as well as a Caesarean birth.
● If the surgical scar was a transverse one.
● If you have been in continuous touch with a supportive practitioner.

In the birth itself you should not have any induction or hormone stimulation, you should be assisted by a midwife continuously, and walk around and move about during labour.

The Birth Itself

Some useful guidelines follow:

Your Companion
Continuous care during birth from a partner or companion has been shown to cut the length of labour, often by half, and lead to fewer Caesareans compared with mothers without such allies.[43] It also leads to less pain and medication,[44] and the quality of the experience is improved. Indeed a PhD thesis on this issue found that 'peak experiences' during childbirth were reported only by women whose husbands were with them.[45] The support is massage, talking, loving, familiarity, getting things and keeping disturbances at bay so that the mother does not have to be on guard. She can concentrate, conserve her energy, relax more and let go.

Familiarity
Personal knicknacks, pictures, your own clothes, flowers or talismans are important within the alien and demeaning hospital environment. They may help you loosen up. My wife stuck a postcard of the vaulted stone entrance archway of University College, Oxford in front of her during one birth. She concentrated so hard on being inside this birth canal that the hospital 'vanished'.

Sustenance
Labour is exhausting. You may need a little nourishment on the way. As obstetricians are crisis-oriented, they have Caesarean-under-general-anaesthetic continually at the back of their minds. So in hospital this nourishment is usually provided in the form of a drip to keep your stomach empty in case of surgery. Refuse the drip. You can have small sips of water or herb tea sweetened with honey without risk, and you can be given a drip later if you really have to have it.

Speeding Things Up
If you are informed that your labour is 'not progressing', your partner should be sceptical, at least initially, and request that you be left alone to get on with it in your own time. If the doctor insists on induction ask if it is absolutely necessary, ask for more time or ask for a second opinion. Meanwhile here are some tricks:

● Walk (especially up and down stairs), squat, change position, move about. This is the best way of getting things going.
● Take a little sustenance as described above.
● Relax yourself completely using slow steady breathing. Concentration on the breath, as in yoga, is effective in aiding the opening of the cervix.
● The brain hormones which control labour can be stimulated by suggestion. In India a grain jar is broken and the grain slowly poured out, or a flower bud is placed by the mother so that her cervix will open as it unfurls. Your partner can take you through guided imagery of opening, releasing and breaking.
● Sexual stimulation can hasten labour, again through the hormones. In Jamaica women are given a man's sweaty shirt to smell.[46] Labour can be initiated and hastened by gently handling the nipples or by bringing another baby to suck.
● Acupuncture is probably the most reliable of the complementary methods for hastening labour. It stimulates the uterus, bringing renewed energy to the whole birth process. Here is an account by a mother whose contractions ceased after 24 hours of labour. The doctor wanted to induce the birth but the mother insisted on calling her acupuncturist. She writes:

'When my acupuncturist arrives I feel calmer. I feel needles making connection. About every five minutes he takes my pulses and slightly turns the needles which are left in. I feel extra surges of energy from those points every time he does another set of manipulations. I begin to feel the increased energy flow centering on my pelvis area, and after 10 or 15 minutes I experience my first contractions . . .'

From an acupuncturist's point of view, there are very precise points involved but it needs experience to select the appropriate points for each case. There are not many acupuncturists as yet in the West who are experienced at assisting delivery. The kind of technique used is illustrated by Jan Resnick, a UK acupuncturist in the case of Chris, whose contractions were weak and intermittent:

'We went on to leave needles in colon 4, stomach 36 and spleen 6 for 30–40 minutes. Chris felt a lot of sensation drawing on her womb, and within 10 minutes contractions began to increase in strength and frequency. Our spirits rose as progress was initiated but within 2 hours everything slowed right down. So we tried a second treatment which included the ear points called "uterus" and "endocrine" plus other points which the Chinese refer to in this context as "promoting labour", "benefitting the uterus", "moving the blood" and "dilating the cervix and facilitating delivery". Chris responded as before, with an impressive surge of energy, stronger contractions and a further opening of her cervix . . . before we knew it we were in transition.'

● Cranial osteopaths claim to be able to hasten and ease labour by gentle manipulation of the base of the skull. For example David Stebbings, a UK osteopath, writes that in overdue cases or in slow labour he can often feel compression and tightness at the base of the skull. Treatment frees this area leaving the mother more relaxed, lighter and more ready to deliver.

Pain

Try to avoid anaesthetics, narcotics and especially tranquillizers. To accept an epidural is a critical and irreversible decision. You can postpone the decision and have an epidural later in the birth anyway, although it is somewhat more difficult. Meanwhile you can try and use more natural methods of pain control including breathing, relaxation imagery and massage. Massage the back firmly during a posterior birth (the baby facing and pressing on the mother's back) and use efflorage – light strokes on the abdomen – for an anterior birth. You will find that at the moment when you cannot bear it one more minute, the birth is almost over – you have reached the top and are going down the other side.

The commonest complementary method of reducing pain is acupuncture. This, with other pain-control methods, is discussed in Chapter 5. If you want to use acupuncture you must find someone who will do it, and request the co-operation of your doctor. Here is one woman's account of her acupuncture experience:

'We reached hospital at 6.30 p.m. At 7.30 the doctor came, examined me and announced I was 4½ centimetres dilated and was not going home without a baby. My husband, Greg, cheered. At 10.30 p.m. the acupuncturist placed the first needle in my left hand, between the thumb and forefinger well up in the crevice that separates them. The needles are so thin that they would more properly be called wires . . . it is barely possible to feel them enter let alone any pain.

Next a needle was placed in each of my calves, then two were placed in each of my feet. They were placed slowly and carefully taking time out during my contractions. During this process I continued to practice Lamaze breathing. The entire procedure took approximately 20 minutes. The relief from the acupuncture occurred at the end of this 20 minute period . . . As soon as the acupuncture took effect, the resident anaesthesiologist asked me to compare contractions. I felt that the next four were reduced in pain by half.'[47]

If you do take painkilling drugs during birth there is not much you can do to prevent the baby receiving them. At least you can be prepared for the baby to be a little slow in feeding and reacting. You can help yourself to overcome any fogginess and dopiness from the drugs by washing them out with plenty of drink, by taking B vitamins together with small nutritious high-protein and low-starch meals, and by taking stimulating herb teas such as ginseng (see Chapter 10).

A Quick Getaway

The hospital is not a particularly conducive place to begin your new relationship, nor to start the rhythms of caring. You can ask for a 24-hour discharge beforehand, provided you do not have six children and the washing up waiting for you. Some hospitals accept the so-called 'domino system' in which you deliver, have a cup of tea and leave, but you must request it beforehand.

Caesarean Section

You may have done your best, and prepared yourself well, but sometimes things do go wrong, and if you are satisfied that a Caesarean is necessary on clear medical grounds, what should you do to reduce the risks? In most cases you will have time to prepare for it. All the recommendations and suggestions given in Chapter 6 on surgery in general and in Chapter 5 on anaesthesia apply here too, and these will help you survive a Caesarian as surgery. You can also get help from special Caesarean preparation classes, from the books described and from Caesarean groups.

It is important for the health of the baby that you only go to the operating theatre *after* natural labour has begun. This reduces the dangers to the foetus of prematurity. Respiratory distress is *several times* less frequent when a Caesarean section is performed after labour has begun.[48]

Ask for a low transverse cut in the abdomen, which is usually hidden after a while by pubic hair, and a transverse cut in the uterus. This cut has much less chance of breaking in a future normal birth than the vertical cut.

Preoperative medication is mostly unnecessary, especially in a Caesarean where every drug compromises the baby to some extent and tranquillizers more than most. Choose a spinal or epidural anaesthetic rather than a general anaesthetic. It has less side effects on both the mother and child, it permits the mother to have contact with the baby straight after the birth, to share the birth with the father and to be more involved. There is evidence that it minimizes any depression and sense of failure. Indeed anything that keeps the mother more in contact with delivery, especially keeping awake for it, will help to prevent later problems of relating to the baby, the birth and herself.[49]

The father can share the procedure, give support, alleviate the sense of helplessness and anxiety and hold the baby soon after birth. It is absurd to think that a strange nurse, with one or two kind words, can replace him. The father can help even if the mother is unconscious during a general anaesthetic: he acts as her eyes and ears during the event. It used to be a fear of obstetricians that fathers at any birth, let alone at a Caesarean, would get in the way, or faint, or sue. This has now been amply disproved and indeed the National Institute of Health now recommends fathers' presence at Caesareans since they found that it helps the mother to recover more quickly.[50]

The best place to start breastfeeding is in the recovery room, immediately after the operation. There is no reason why you should not start straight away, although the drugs may make it more difficult. Nevertheless it is better there than after the anaesthetic has worn off and the pain begins. If the colostrum (the clear liquid that precedes milk) does not flow and the baby does not suck so readily, do not see it as another 'failure' – it is more likely to be due to the drugs and the answer is to try again occasionally.

You should choose a hospital for your Caesarean which encourages breastfeeding, and has a reputation for flexibility and understanding. You should also make sure of 24-hour visiting by the father, a great deal of information from the staff, and a room with other Caesarean mothers.

Protecting your Baby from Medical Side Effects

You can assume that whatever you experience the baby will receive too, in good measure. What can you do to protect the baby from the stresses of treatment?

One of the best ways is *breastfeeding on demand*. Even if the baby seems sleepy and sucks weakly you can express a few drops of colostrum. If it is in special care your milk is vital. A new study has proved that fresh breast milk is the best medicine for newborns after difficult births. Babies in special care receiving fresh milk had half as many infections as those receiving pasteurized human milk or human milk and formula.[51]

Do not allow substitutes such as formula or sugar-water. These make it more difficult to begin breast-feeding. They do not provide the baby with the protection and immunity it needs straight after birth. When the nurses tried to persuade us to give sugar water to one of our babies they said it was because the hospital air conditioning dried up the babies and they needed the extra liquid. So we asked for fresh air instead. A drugged baby, arriving after a violent medical birth, needs extra contact, nourishment, and warmth which breast-feeding on demand can provide. Breast-feeding rhythms can be established later.

There is a major problem with breast-feeding: the torture of *cracked nipples*. This arises from poor technique; the hospital should show you how to tease the baby with the nipple so that it sucks with mouth agape, taking in the areola and not sucking on the nipple itself. If you do get cracked nipples use wheat germ oil to prevent inflammation and heal the cracks rather than the cream the hospital will provide.

Whenever you take any drug it will enter your bloodstream within minutes and leave within hours. Any drugs that are necessary should be taken straight after a feed so that much of it will have gone by the time the next feed comes round. This is obviously something to plan carefully with your doctor.

As drugs pass to the baby, so do *vitamins*. You can help your newborn after a medicalized birth by giving it vitamins in your milk. You should take B vitamins, and vitamin E and C in the dosages described in Chapter 4. This is in addition to the vitamins the hospital will give the newborn. Doctors recently reported in the *British Medical Journal* that vitamin E supplements (unheard of by most paediatricians) given to premature babies improve their chances of survival.[52] Tell them.

There are *psychological side effects* of special care which, though subtle, can be more profound than the physical ones because they last longer. They arise from the disconnections between mother and child. Try to avoid hospitals where newborns are routinely sent to special care after a Caesarean. If your newborn is in special care for real medical necessity, be its nurse. Do everything for it yourself. Express milk for it, feed it, even switch on the machines for it.

When you get home, and the baby is safely nested consider what you can do to remove any scars of a medicalized birth from both of you. Difficult or traumatic births, especially by forceps, can leave tensions in the baby which make it fretful. Small babies respond well to homeopathic treatment for symptoms which may have arisen from drug side effects. Try a homeopath first. Osteopathy, especially cranial osteopathy, can help release these tensions, calm the baby and soften the 'body memory' of the birth. Osteopaths have found that mechanical distortions of the top of the chest and neck area can be caused by forceps and difficult births. It can disturb the nerves which control breathing, leading to childhood asthma. They are sometimes able to correct the mechanical distortions and cure the asthma.

Massage is also useful. Use thumb and forefinger to gently massage the limbs and back. There are instructions in the books by the French natural childbirth pioneer F. Leboyer. Use a little inert oil such as almond or olive but not essential oils of herbs, which may be toxic. Touch, contact and your love can do a great deal to restore a peaceful connection with your baby, letting the healing happen by itself.

REFERENCES

1. Brooks, D. *Naturebirth,* Heinemann, London (1985).
2. Shearer, M. H. *Birth and Fam. Journal,* 6 119–125 (1974).
3. Mendelsohn, M. *Malepractice,* Contemporary Books, Chicago (1981).
4. Quoted in ref. 1.
5. Howard, F. M. *Obstetrics and Gynaecology,* 11 318 (1958); Newton, N. and Newton, M., *Obstetrics and Gynaecology,* 15 28 (1960); Mengert, quoted in ref. 3.
6. *Internat. Childbirth Education Assoc.,* Special Report, Vol. II (1972).
7. *Lancet* 2, 1183 (1974).
8. Gosh. A. and Hudson F. P. *Lancet,* 823 (1977).
9. Field, H. *Obstetrics and Gynaecology,* 15 476 (1960).
10. Sims, D. G. & Neligan, G. A. *Br. J. Obst. Gyn.,* 82 863–867 (1975); Jeffaries, M. J. *Ibid,* 84 452–455 (1977); Lange, A. P. *et. al., Lancet,* 1 991–4 (1982).
11. Knepp, N. B. *et al, Lancet,* 1 1150–2 (1982); Mendiola *et al, Anaesthesia and Analgesia,* 61 32–35 (1982); Singhi, S. *et al Lancet,* 2 335–6 (1982).
12. Garcia, J. *et al, Birth,* 12 79–85 (1985).
13. Caldeyro-Barcia, R. *Birth Fam. J.,* 2 5–14 (1974).
14. Macdonald, D. *et al Am. J. Obst. Gynaecol.,* 152 524–539 (1985); Bantal H. D. and Thacker, S. B. *Birth Fam. J.,* 6 232 (1979).
15. Kimball, *et al, Pacific Counties Obst. Gynaecol. Society Reports,* October 1980.
16. Gintzler, A. R. *Science,* 210 193 (1980).
17. Clark, A. J. and Affonzo, D. *Childbearing, A Nursing Perspective,* Philadelphia, Davis (1976).
18. Hellman, L. and Pritchard, J. *Williams Obstetrics,* 14th Edition, N.Y. (1971).
19. Kron, *et al, Paediatrics,* 37 1012 (1966); Stechler, *Science,* 144 315 (1964).
20. Bowes, W. A. *Monographs of the Society for Research on Child Development,* 35 no. 4 (1970).

21. Richards, M. P. M. *Feeding and Early Growth of the Mother-Child Relationship,* Basel, S. Karger (1973); Richards, M. P. M. New Scientist, P. 820 (28 March 1974).
22. Brackbill, Y. 'Obstetric Medication and Infant Development', In: Osofsky (ed.) *Handbook of Infant Development,* New York, Wiley, (1971).
23. Vasicky, A. *Obst. & Gynecol.,* **38** 500 (71); Rosefsky, J. & Petersiel, M. *N. Eng. J. Med.,* **278** 530 (68).
24. Cree, J. *B.M.J.,* **4** 251 (1973).
25. D.H.S.S. Report on Confidential Enquiries into Maternal Deaths in England and Wales 1970–2; Report on Health & Social Subjects, No. 11 (1975). For the U.S., See Petitti, D. *et al, Am. J. Obstet. Gynaecol.,* **133** 391 (1978).
26. Editorial, *Brit. Med. J.,* 978–9, (24 April 1976)
27. Morewood, G. A. *et al, Obstet. Gynaecol.,* **42** 589 (1973).
28. Marieskind, H. I. *An Evaluation of Caesarian Section in the U.S.,* Office of the Assistant Secretary for Planning & Education/Health, Washington, U.S. Govt. Printing Office (1979).
29. Merrill, B. S. and Gibbs C. E. *Obst. Gynaecol.,* **52,** 50 (78); Donnelly, J. P. and Franzoni K. T. *Obst. Gynaecol.,* **29** 871 (1967).
30. Baskell, T. F. *Canadian Med. Assoc. J.,* **118** 1019 (1978); Hibbard, L. T. *Am. J. Obstet. Gynaecol.,* **125** 798 (1976).
31. See *Obstet. and Gynaecol.,* (August 1984).
32. Butler, N. R. and Alberman, E. D. *Perinatal Problems,* London, Publisher unknown (1960).
33. Harrison, R. F. *et al, Brit. Med. J.,* **288** 1971–5 (1980).
34. Sleep, J. *et al, Brit. Med. J.,* **289** 587–590 (1980).
35. See ref. 26 of Chap. 6.
36. Richards, M. P. M. *Birth and Fam. J.,* **7** 225–233 (1980); Rumeau Rouquette, C., *et al, Naitre en France, Dix ans d'evolution,* Paris, Editions INSERM (1984).
37. Chamberlain, R. *et al, British Births,* 1970, Vol. 1, London, Heinemann Medical (1975).
38. Brooks, D. (ref. 1); Kitzinger, S. *The New Good Birth Guide,* London Penguin, (1983); Stanway, P. and A. *Choices in Childbirth* Pan (1984); Ibid, *Baby and Child Book,* London Pan (1984); Odent, M. *Birth Reborn,* London Souvenir (1984); Noble, E. *Childbirth with Insight,* Boston, Houghton Mifflin, (1984).
39. Richards, M. P. M. *J. Maternal and Child Health,* (September 1979).
40. O'Leary, J. A. *Obstet. Gynaecol.,* **53** 341 (1979); Collea, J. V. *et al, Am. J. Obstet. Gynaecol.,* **131** 186 (1978).
41. Fall, O. *et al, Obstet. Gynaecol* **53** 713 (1979).
42. Shy, K. K. *et al, Am. J. Obstet. Gynaecol.,* **139** 123 (1981).
43. Sosa, R. *et al, New Eng. J. Med.* **303** 597–600 (1980).
44. Henneborn, W. S. and Cogan, R. *J. Psychosomatic Res.,* **19** 215–222 (1975).
45. Tanzer, D. *The Psychology of Pregnancy and Childbirth: an Investigation of Natural Childbirth,* Brandeis University, Ph. D. Thesis (1967).

46. Bates, B. and Newman Turner, A. *Birth,* **12** 29–35 (1985).
47. *Birth and Family Journal,* **1**, 16.
48. Maisels, M. J. *et al, J. American Med. Assoc.,* **238** 206 (1977).
49. Cohen, N. *Birth and Family J.,* **4** 114 (1977).
50. U.S. Dept. Health and Human Services: *Caesarian Childbirth, Report of a Consensus Development Conference,* NIH Pub. No. 82-2067 (1981).
51. Narayanan, I., *et al, Lancet,* **2**, 1111-3 (1984).
52. *British Medical J.,* **287** 81 (1983).

CHAPTER 13

Risks to the Healthy:
Vaccinations and Dentistry

Which Vaccinations are Worth It?: A Holistic Perspective

An holistically minded parent would want to give only those vaccinations which are highly effective, which prevent real risk of life-threatening disease, and which do not have unacceptable side effects. Others will be seen as bearing too much risk for insufficient benefit. They will be assumed to result from medical oversell without really knowing the full long-term consequences. Vaccination is an area of potentially explosive confrontation between the public and the medical profession, because their interests here are more sharply divergent than when the profession comes to the aid of the sick. The public will not accept the pain of seeing a healthy baby today become a vaccine-damaged baby tomorrow. But the doctors are under pressure from Government, from the profession and from the pharmaceutical industry to vaccinate as much as possible. After all, do not vaccinations protect the public as a whole from contagious disease? This puts considerable pressure on parents to vaccinate their children as a social duty.

However all is not as it seems. Firstly some diseases, such as measles or whooping cough would still exist in the UK even if every single child were vaccinated. Although, naturally, without any vaccination programme the disease would increase. Second, there is strong evidence that many contagious diseases such as T.B. are decreased far more by sanitation and public health than by vaccination. Third, vaccinations can make disease much worse when it does occur. Polio is a very mild disease in Egypt, where there is little vaccination, crippling less than 1% of cases. It is a severe disease if it occurs in England, crippling the majority of cases.[1]

Holistically minded parents will want to make a different kind of calculation than the one usually made for them by the doctor. They will know that infectious diseases such as measles or whooping cough are more serious if the child is poorly nourished and generally unhealthy. Therefore they would prefer to feed the child and take the risk of a 1:100,000 chance of death from whooping cough rather than receive a 1:130,000 risk of death and an additional risk of brain damage from whooping cough vaccine. Furthermore anyone who has had contact with complementary medicine today, or even the more natural-minded family doctors of 40 years ago, will know that it is better to catch the usual children's diseases such as measles or mumps, and get over them properly, than to suppress them by vaccination or other medical means. Complementary practitioners, especially homeopaths, know that this suppression weakens the immunity and may be to blame for *some* of the terrible chronic disease burden of Western man in later life, e.g. multiple sclerosis, arthritis, asthma, allergies and cancer. A new study, providing dramatic support for this view, appeared unexpectedly in the *Lancet*. The State Serum Institute in Copenhagen found that those children who had some immunity to measles (from vaccination or symptomatically healed measles) but did not have full measles with rash, developed more skin diseases, bone diseases and certain cancers in later life.[2]

Which vaccinations are worth it? This is a very difficult decision and can only be based on assessment. I give below what I allow for my own children and why. It represents my own 'Get the Best and Leave the Rest' position. It is unwise to be dogmatic.

1: Vaccination Worth While

Disease	Considerations
Polio	Disease risk is considerable, vaccination limits the disease in society and has little risk. Highly effective.
Diphtheria	As above.
Smallpox	Last naturally caught case in the UK in 1971. Not necessary unless required for travel, but then as above.
Tetanus	Highly effective and harmless. It is available with diphtheria only (DT), or with diphtheria and whooping cough (DPT).
Rubella (German measles)	Only if a girl at puberty missed catching it previously (because of possible risk in pregnancy).
Typhoid, typhus and yellow fever	If going to affected area or if required by law. More or less effective.
Hepatitis	Worthwhile only if in high-risk situation.

2: Vaccination Not Worthwhile

Disease	Considerations
Whooping cough	Risks are greater than the risks from the disease provided child receives good nutrition and care (see below).
Measles, mumps	Preferable to catch the disease and get over it with good care. There is evidence of damage to immunity with these vaccines[2,3] and other rare but serious effects.
BCG (anti-tuberculosis)	Not very effective. Tuberculosis is easily preventible by good nutrition, care and hygiene.
Rubella (German measles)	Make sure your child joins German measles infected children and gets the disease. See measles, mumps, and rubella (table 1).
Cold and Influenza	These are largely ineffective[4] and there are occasional side effects.[5]
Cholera	Only partly effective and of brief duration, but leads to carelessness. Does not protect families of cholera sufferers.

Whooping Cough Vaccine

A word about pertussis, whooping cough vaccine, which has been the subject of intense debate. Most children have been vaccinated with pertussis, a few receiving side effects such as rash, fever, screaming, and earaches, and more rarely high fever and convulsions. Long-term but infrequent side effects include allergies, asthma, fits, sensory disorders and mental retardation. A study at UCLA found pertussis was responsible for some 15% of all sudden infant 'cot deaths'. This is worrying enough, particularly because the risks of serious or permanent damage (usually brain damage) resulting from the vaccine are, or were, as great as from the disease itself.[6] However some doctors and researchers feel that the risks are very much greater but unknown. They are buried among the large numbers of children diagnosed every year as mentally retarded and the millions of all children in the category of 'hyperactive' or 'learning disability'. The evidence for this is from interviews of parents, a kind of research that medicine rarely carries out.[7] Parents sometimes notice behavioural changes after vaccinations that doctors miss. Indeed the long-term results of pertussis vaccination have not been assessed, despite warnings. The effects of the newer vaccine, which is meant to be better, are similarly unknown.

At the same time the protection given by whooping cough vaccine is not great, and children can still catch the disease and pass it on.[8]

Both the disease and the vaccination are more serious in the very young. For these reasons I would not vaccinate my children with this vaccine, and similar arguments apply to the others in the second group. Instead I would rely on lengthy breastfeeding to cover the early vulnerable period of their life, followed by good nutrition, fresh air and minimal drugs to husband their immunity thereafter.

One family we spoke to had refused whooping cough vaccine for their baby, who then subsequently had actually caught whooping cough. What they say is interesting:

> We decided not to vaccinate our son because we didn't feel the risks were fully known. Friends had told us that their children had changed after vaccination and we were afraid of subtle and perhaps unmeasurable consequences. Well, our boy caught whooping cough at one and a half years. It really is a terrible disease – he was coughing pitifully for eight weeks and continued to cough, though less frequently, into the next winter until we took him to Spain for a holiday. But he got over it himself. It was his fight, his body, his immunity. We watched his own defences rise to the occasion, with our help. We would rather have had it this way. For if, as parents, we had allowed the injection of something into the child that had caused even the slightest damage, we would have felt far more guilty. We could never have lived with it.

Preventing Vaccination Side Effects

When you have vaccinations of any kind, here are some suggestions on how to minimise the chances of side effects appearing.

The main method is to make sure the child is healthy and well when he or she is vaccinated. Do not vaccinate if the child or baby is crying more than usual, off colour or ill, especially with a fever, or has a generally depressed immunity.

Do not give too many different vaccinations all at once 'to get them over with'. It may be too much for the unformed immune system to cope with. The child should fully get over one before having the next.

Do not have whooping cough vaccination, and minimise the other vaccinations, if the child or your family has a history of convulsions, neurological disorders or allergies, especially eczema.

If the child reacts badly to the first dose of a vaccine it is an indication that it may have more serious side effects later. Watch the child very carefully after vaccination, and tell your doctor about anything beyond some general fretfulness.

Holistically oriented doctors often give vitamin C in a dose of ½gm or more along with vaccinations, especially measles.

Homeopathy is the only system within complementary medicine

which has tried to develop remedies against vaccination side effects. This arises from a deeply held conviction among traditional homeopaths than any vaccination is damaging to general health and immunity. Therefore vaccinations are to some extent regarded as conditions to be treated. The usual method is to give homeopathic remedies that mimic the symptom picture that would occur with vaccination side effects. For example after German measles vaccination Pulsatilla 30 is given as antidote and after BCG (anti-tuberculosis), Silica 30.

Homeopathy also has its own kind of protection against infectious diseases as a harmless substitute for conventional vaccinations. These are inactivated disease agencies (nosodes) which are superficially similar to the vaccinations but vastly more dilute. For example the Pertussin 30 nosode is given every three weeks throughout autumn and winter to protect against whooping cough, or Morbillinum 30 to protect against measles. Additional remedies are taken when exposed to infection.

Dental Amalgam and Metal Toxicity

The Chinese invented mercury amalgam for filling teeth in the 6th century, and it was reinvented in the 18th century. Mercury is highly toxic. There have always been occasional worries about its use: in 1840 the American Society of Dental Surgeons made its members sign that they would never put amalgam in patients' mouths. Today the dental establishment sees mercury toxicity as a problem for dentists, not for patients.[9] However mercury is continually released from fillings by corrosion[10], by chewing[11], and by electrical microcurrents caused by different metals in the mouth.[12] This mercury enters the blood stream or is inhaled, and some may even work its way along nerves. Mercury has been found in the brain in amounts proportional to the number of amalgam fillings in the mouth.

A group of doctors and dentists, as well as homeopaths, say that mercury amalgam can cause sleep disturbance, depression, headaches, fatigue and debility, neuromuscular problems, multiple sclerosis, neuralgia, mouth ulcers, skin problems and asthma.[13] This is based on cases they have seen which have cleared up when the amalgams are removed. There is little support from research as yet, but there is some evidence that mercury amalgams adversely affect the immunity, which could indeed account for a variety of health problems.[14]

It would be imprudent to support a general scare about amalgams. Most people have them without problems. Yet there may be some people who become sensitive or sensitized to mercury and you should be aware of the possibility that mercury could gradually cause side effects.

In case you have one of the above problems that doesn't go away and doesn't seem to result from other causes, naturopaths and many holistic doctors can carry out tests which indicate abnormal sensitivity to mercury or mercury toxicity. Treatment involves clearing the body of heavy metal toxicity by a restricted diet and by the consumption of nutritional supplements that capture the metals in the body: vitamin C, selenium, cysteine, glutathione, zinc and magnesium. Blood-purifying herbs and herbs to to help the elimination of the metals can be given. Treatment is monitored by mercury testing in the urine. Homeopaths can give homeopathic antidotes.

If abnormal sensitivity to mercury is shown the amalgams should be removed and replaced with newer non-mercury composite fillings. However some holistic doctors and dentists would only remove fillings that seem unstable and release mercury, leaving others. The removal of amalgams itself creates toxic mercury vapour so it must be done carefully.

Consider using newer non-mercury white composites for your future fillings on your back as well as your front teeth, especially if you tend to be allergic or sensitive to toxins. Holistic dentists can be found these days who will bear all this in mind when treating your teeth.

REFERENCES

1. McKeown, T. *The Role of Medicine: Dream, Mirage or Nemesis*, Nuffield Provincial Hospital Trust, London (1976); Howe, G. M. *Man Environment and Disease in Britain*, Harmondsworth, Middlesex, Pelican (1976).
2. Ronne, T. *Lancet,* **1** 1–4 (1985).
3. Buttram, H. E. and Hoffman, J. C. *Vaccinations and Immune Malfunctions*, Humanitarian Press, PA. (1982); Wilkins, J. and Wherle, P. *J. Paedriatrics,* 865–869 (June 1979).
4. Smith, J. *Lancet* **2** 330 (1974).
5. *The Guardian* (7 June 1979).
6. Steward, G. T. *Brit. Med. J.,* **287** 287–8 (1983).
7. Coulter, H. L. and Fisher, B. L. *DPT–A Shot in the Dark*, Harcourt Brace, Jovanovitch, NY & London (1983).
8. Steward, G. T. *Lancet,* **1** 234–237 (1977).
9. White *et al, J. Am. Dental Soc.,* **92** 1204–1207 (1976).
10. Derand, *et al, Scandinavian J. Dent. Res.,* **91** 55–60 (1983).
11. Gay, D. *et al, Lancet,* **1** 985–6 (1978).

12. Wakai, *J. Am. Dental Assoc.,* **23** 1000–1006 (1936).
13. Hoffer, A., *J. Orthomolecular Psychiatry,* 13 (1984).
14. Eggleston, D. W., *J. Prosthetic Dentistry,* **51**, 617–622 (1984).

Appendix

Self-help Groups

Action for the Victims of Medical
Accidents (AVMA),
24 Southwark Street,
London SE1 1TY.
Tel: 01-403 4744

Active Birth Movement, The,
55, Dartmouth Park Road,
London NW5

Arthritic Association,
122 Three Bridges Road, Crawley,
W. Sussex. Tel: 0293 22041

Association for Improvements in the
Maternity Services (AIMS),
163 Liverpool Road, London N1 0RF.
Tel: 01-278 5628

Association of Parents of Vaccine
Damaged Children,
2 Church Street, Shipston-on-Stour,
Warwickshire, CV36 4AP.
Tel: 0608 61595

Back-Up (An information service for
cancer patients)
121–123 Charterhouse Street,
London EC1. Tel: 01-608 1661

Birth Rights,
Yvonne Baginsky, 2 Forth Street,
Edinburgh, EH1 3LD

British Diabetic Association,
10 Queen Anne Street, London
W1M 0BD. Tel: 01-323 1531

Caesarian Support Group of
Cambridge,
Ann Watson, 7 Green Street,
Willingham, Cambs. CB4 5JA.
Tel: 0954 60630

Cancer Contact,
Hon. Organiser: 0444 454043
Hon. Treasurer and Support Section:
0444 413055

Cancer Help Centre,
Grove House, Cornwallis Grove,
Clifton, Bristol BA8 4PG.
Tel: 0272 743216

Cancerlink,
46 Pentonville Road,
London N1 9HF. Tel: 01-833 2451

Family Heart Association,
(Familial Hypercholesterolaemia and
Familial Hyperlipidaemia
Association),
P.O. Box 116, Kidlington, Oxford
OX5 1DT

Guillain Barre Syndrome,
45 Parkfield Road, Ruskington,
Sleaford, Lincs. NG34 9HT.
Tel: 0526 832046

Heart to Heart,
P.O. Box 7, High Street, Pershore,
Worcestershire.

Hysterectomy Support Group,
Judy Vaughan, Rivendell, Warren
Way, Lower Heswall, Wirral,
Merseyside. Tel: 051 342 3167

Intractable Pain Society of Great
Britain and Ireland,
Pain Relief Clinic, Basingstoke
District Hospital, Aldermaston Road,
Basingstoke, Hants. RG24 9NA.
Tel: 0256 473202

Justice for *All* Vaccine Damaged
Children,
Enid and Ivor Needs, Erins Cottage,
Fussells Buildings, Whiteway Road,
St. George, Bristol BS5 7QY.
Tel: 0272 557818

Leukaemia Care Society,
P.O. Box 82, Exeter, Devon
EX2 5LP. Tel: 0592 218514

Lupus Group,
6 Grosvenor Crescent, London
SW1X 7ER. Tel: 01-235 0902/5

Mastectomy Association,
26 Harrison Street, off Gray's Inn
Road, London WC1H 8JG.
Tel: 01-837 0908

Mind (National Association for
Mental Health),
22 Harley Street, London W1N 2ED.
Tel: 01-637 0741

NAC (New Approaches to Cancer),
c/o The Seekers Trust, The Close,
Addington Park, Maidstone, Kent
ME19 5BL. Tel: 0732 848336

National Association for Colitis and
Crohn's Disease (NACC)
98A London Road, St. Albans, Herts.
AL1 1NX.

National Association for the Welfare
of Children in Hospital (NAWCH),
Argyle House, 29–31 Euston Road,
London NW1 2SD. Tel: 01-833 2041

National Childbirth Trust,
9 Queensborough Terrace, London
W2 3TB. Tel: 01-221 3833

National Federation of Kidney
Patients' Associations,
Acorn Lodge, Woodsetts, Worksop,
Notts. S81 8AT. Tel: 0909 562703

Opren Action Group,
13 Carlton Close, Debenham,
Norfolk. Tel: 0362 67483

Psoriasis Association,
7 Milton Street, Northampton,
NN2 7JG. Tel: 0604 711129

Renal Society,
64 South Hill Park, London
NW3 2SJ. Tel: 01-794 9479

Steroid-Action Aid-Group,
67 Hammersmith Grove, London
W6 0NE. Tel: 01-748 3589

TRANX (Tranquillizer Recovery and
New Existence),
Ms. Joan Jerome, 17 Peel Road,
Wealdstone, Middlesex.
Tel: 01-427 2065

Women's Health Concern,
WHC Flat, 17 Earls Terrace, London
W8 6LP. Tel: 01-602 6669

Women's Health Information Centre,
52/54 Featherstone Street, London
EC1Y 8RT. Tel: 01-251 6580

For further information see:

Grann, R.,
The Health Information Handbook,
Gower Street, London (1986)

or contact:

The Patients Association,
18 Charing Cross Road,
London WC2 0HR.
Tel: 01-240 0671

The College of Health,
18 Victoria Park Square,
London E2 9PF

Complementary Medical Organizations

Association for New Approaches to
Cancer,
231 Kensal Road, London W10 5DB.
Tel: 01-969 1684

Bristol Cancer Help Centre,
Grove House, Cornwallis Grove,
Clifton, Bristol BS8 4PG.
Tel: 0272 743216

British Acupuncture Association and
Register,
34 Alderney Street,
London SW1V 4EU.
Tel: 01-834 3353/1012

British Alliance of Healing
Associations,
23 Nutcroft Grove, Fetcham,
Leatherhead, Surrey. Tel: 0372 373241

British Association for Holistic
Health,
179 Gloucester Place, London
NW1 6DX. Tel: 01-262 5299

British Dental Society for Clinical
Nutrition,
Flat 5, 30 Harley Street, London
W1N 1AB.

British Holistic Medical Association,
179 Gloucester Place, London
NW1 6LX. Tel: 01-262 5299

British Homeopathic Association,
27a Devonshire Street, London
W1N 1RJ. Tel: 01-935 2163

British Medical Acupuncture Society,
67–69 Chancery Lane, London
WC2A 1AF

British Naturopathic and Osteopathic
Association,
Frazer House, 6 Netherhall Gardens,
London NW3 5RR. Tel: 01-435 8728

British Society of Medical and Dental
Hypnosis,
42 Links Road, Ashtead, Surrey
KT21 2HJ. Tel: 01-277 3522

British Society for Nutritional
Medicine,
4 Museum Street, York YO1 2ES

Centre for Autogenic Training,
101 Harley Street, London W1N 1DF.
Tel: 01-935 1811

Centre for Yoga Studies,
48 Devonshire Buildings, Bath
BA2 4SU. Tel: 0225 26327

College of Health,
18 Victoria Park Square, London
E2 9PF.

Faculty of Homeopathy,
The Royal London Homeopathic
Hospital, Great Ormond Street,
London WC1N 3HR. Tel: 01-837 3091
Ext. 72

Friends Fellowship of Healing,
Lilian Palmer, 5 Old Manor Close,
Ifield, Crawley, RH11 0HQ.

The Holistic Council for Cancer,
Runnings Park, Croft Bank, West
Malvern, Worcester WR14 4BP.
Tel: 06845 65286

Holistic Pharmacists Association,
50 St. Gabriels Road, London
NW2 4SA. Tel: 01-452 0371

Homeopathic Hospitals
The Royal London Homeopathic
Hospital, Great Ormond Street,
London WC1N 3HR.
The Glasgow Homeopathic Hospital,
1000 Great Western Road, Glasgow
G12 0RN.
Outpatients Department, 5 Lynedoch
Road, Glasgow C3.
Outpatients Clinic, Baillieston Health
Institute, Buchanan Street, Baillieston,
Glasgow.
Liverpool Clinic, The Mossley Hill
Hospital, Park Avenue, Liverpool
L18 8BU.
The Bristol Homeopathic Hospital,
Cotham Road, Cotham, Bristol
BS6 6JU.
Tunbridge Wells Homeopathic
Hospital, Church Road, Tunbridge
Wells, Kent.

International Stress and Tension
Control Soceity,
The Priory Hospital, Priory Lane,
Roehampton, London SW15 5JJ

Kushi Institute,
188 Old Street, London EC1.
Tel: 01-251 4076

London and Counties Society of
Physiologists,
100 Waterloo Road, Blackpool
FY4 1AW. Tel: 0253 403548

London School of Aromatherapy,
P.O. Box 780, London NW6 5EQ.

The McCarrison Society,
24 Paddington Street, London
W1H 4DR

National Association of Hypnotists
and Psychotherapists,
Marine Villa, Ferry Road, Earlsferry,
Elie, Fife KY9 1AJ. Tel: 0333 330364

National Council of Psychotherapists
and Hypnotherapy Registry,
Stream Cottage, Wish Hill,
Willingdon, E. Sussex BN20 9HQ.
Tel: 0323 501540

National Federation of Spiritual
Healers,
Old Manor Farm Studio, Church
Street, Sunbury-on-Thames, Middlesex
TW16 6RG. Tel: 0932 783164

Natural Health Network, 51 Rodney
Road, Cheltenham GL50 7HX.
Tel: 0242 25437

National Institute of Medical
Herbalists Ltd.,
41 Hatherley Road, Winchester
SO22 6RR

New Approaches to Cancer,
c/o The Seekers Trust, The Close
Addington Park, Maidstone, Kent
ME19 5BL
Tel: 0732 848336

Nutrition Association,
24 Harcourt House, 19 Cavendish
Square, London W1M 0AB

Register of Chinese Herbal Medicine,
c/o Wendy Owen, 138 Prestbury
Road, Cheltenham GLS2 2DP

Relaxation for Living,
Dunesk, 29 Burwood Park Road,
Walton-on-Thames, Surrey
KT12 5LH. Tel: 09322 27826

Relaxation Society,
St. Mary Woolnoth Church, Lombard
Street, London EC3V 9AN.
Tel: 01-626 9701

School of Hypnosis and Advanced
Psychotherapy,
Registrar, 28 Finsbury Park Road,
London N4 2JX. Tel: 01-359 6991

Shiatsu Society, The,
19 Langside Park, Kilbarchan,
Renfrewshire PA10 2EP.
Tel: 05057 4657

Society of Advanced Psychotherapists
and Parapsychologists,
c/o SHAP, 28 Finsbury Park Road,
London N4 2JX. Tel: 01-226 6963

Society of Homeopaths Ltd.,
59 Norfold House Road, London
SW16

Spiritualists' National Union,
General Secretary, Britten House,
Stansted Hall, Stansted Mountfitchet,
Essex CM24 80D. Tel: 0279 812705

Traditional Acupuncture Society,
11 Grange park, Stratford upon Avon,
Warwickshire CV37 6XH.
Tel: 0789 298798

Vegetarian Society,
Parkdale, Dunham Road, Altrincham,
Cheshire WA14 4QG.
Tel: 061 928 0793

Index

abdominal foetal electocardiograph 213
acne 178
acupuncture 3–4, 65, 135, 206; anaesthesia 76–7, 81–3; in hospital 56; immune support 139, 147; obstetric 220–1, 223–4; scar treatment 8, 85, 108–9; training in 10; treatment of drug side effects 185, 187–9, 198–9
adaptogenic remedies 138
adenoids 17, 91
adrenal glands 198–200, 205
adriamycin 133
AIDS virus 23, 26
air ionizers 47–8
alcohol 16, 170, 183
Alexander technique 10
alginates 136, 179
allergies 5, 8, 64
aloe vera 69, 134–5, 180, 196, 202
alternative medicine: see complementary medicine
alternative treatment centres 120
amino acids 32–3, 67, 86, 135
anaesthesia 76–86, 92; by acupuncture 76–7, 81–3; alternatives to 76–7; breathing 79–80; in childbirth 213–15; and hypnosis 80–1; preparation for 78–81; risks 78; side effects 78, 82
anaesthetists 97
analgesics 84, 173
anger 81
angiography 24
anorexia 129
antacids 13–14, 65, 71, 173
antibiotics 17, 143, 146, 176, 193–7; antifungal 145; avoiding 195; effect on digestion 64–5; side effects 5, 59, 174–5, 193–7

anticlotting 106
antidepressants 185–8; and diet 186; side effects 13–14, 145, 173, 176, 185–8; withdrawal 186, 187
anti-inflammatory drugs 176
antioxidants 132
antipsychotics 188–91
anti-radiation pill 32
anxiety 6, 104, 122, 180; in hospital 49–50; post-operative 104; pre-operative 79, 98–102
appendix removal 17, 90–1
appetite loss 179
arnica 70, 107–8
aromatherapy 107
aromatic spices 106
arthritis 12, 63, 200, 201, 205
aspirin 156, 165, 168, 205–6
asthma 228, 235
astragalus 137–8
astringents 70
Ativan 185
autogenics 85, 147
Autogenic Training (AT) 53–4

bach flower remedies 107–8, 199
back operations 91
back pain 12, 198
bacteria 64–5, 193–4
barbiturates 77
barium 28–9
bean curd 61
bedsores 66, 69–70
bedwetting 185
β-blockers 172, 205
bioflavonoids 32, 68, 110–11
biopsy 26, 91, 98
bleomycin 133
blood clots 93
blood pressure 23, 24, 72, 150; drug treatment 1, 5, 158, 159, 172, 202–5; herbal treatment 7